Sexuality and
Birth Control
in
Social and
Community Work

Elphis Christopher

Sexuality and Birth Control
in
Social and
Community Work

Temple Smith · London

First published in Great Britain in 1980
by Maurice Temple Smith Ltd
37 Great Russell Street, London WC1

© Elphis Christopher 1980
ISBN 0 85117 183 4

Typeset by Mason & Weldon Ltd
in Journal Roman Medium

Printed in Great Britain
by A. Wheaton & Co Ltd, Exeter

Dedication

To my mother and father, who were both the eldest of large poor families and who were immigrants.

To my husband Donald and our three daughters Helen, Cara, and Elisabeth.

Finally to my patients, particularly the women of the Haringey Domiciliary Family Planning Service, who have taught me so much.

Contents

Acknowledgements

I should like to thank above all Ms Kathleen von Koch and her daughter Andrée for all their help and encouragement. Ms von Koch managed to decipher my deplorable handwriting and type my manuscripts with such patience.

I should also like to thank Ms Juliet Cheetham and Mr Philip Pestell who both read the first draft and made numerous helpful suggestions.

Thank you, too, to Ms Pinsker of the FPA Book Centre and all those well-wishers too numerous to mention individually, both professional and lay, who after hearing me talk (perhaps in an effort to get me to stop!) told me that I should write a book. I have taken the hint and hope they will be pleased with the result.

Finally to my publisher Maurice Temple Smith who has been so encouraging, positive and helpful when I was so full of doubts.

Preface

Like many doctors, I received little education on human sexuality and, indeed, was not particularly concerned about this apart from having vague feelings that sex was fun and should be enjoyed. I did receive some instruction on family planning, though without it leaving much impression.

In 1966 when I did my family planning training it was less out of interest than due to the influence of a friend, a woman doctor, who suggested doing family planning clinics as a way of 'keeping one's hand in' while bringing up a family.

However, once I started to work regularly in family planning clinics and, particularly, when I started doing domiciliary family planning I became aware that there was much more to family planning than prescribing pills and fitting coils and caps. One was involved in a crucial area of a person's life, where present decisions could have profound future consequences not only for that person but for the partner and existing and, as yet, unborn children. It became challenging and moving to be part of that decision-making process. It was (and is) satisfying to help couples plan and space their children and to feel that a child is wanted for himself. Sadly, I became aware that pregnancies and children could be used as pawns, to gratify immature needs, to bolster self-esteem, to provide reassurance about masculinity and femininity, to punish or control a partner or parents and to give a purpose to lives that seemed to have no other function or meaning. I learned how widespread were sexual and marital difficulties and how these influenced the use and choice of contraception. Further, that disgust with sex, uncertainties about the self and the relationship led to the erratic use of contraception and unwanted pregnancy. I discovered that often very little discussion took place between a couple about sex or contraception or about the decision to have a child. I met much ignorance and embarrassment about sex and a lack of concern about family planning, not only among the disadvantaged but among professional colleagues and saw how this prevented help being sought and given.

I became aware of young people's needs and how society made it difficult for the young to make responsible decisions about their sexuality by both stimulating sexual interest and then denying its existence. Then there was the desperation of the infertile and those who wanted an abortion. The irony inherent in that situation was inescapable and had to be coped with. I was occasionally forced into somewhat devious behaviour on behalf of women wanting an abortion whose GP and/or local gynaecologist were anti-abortion. I learned to respect the woman's decision about abortion. It was (and is) invariably a rational and sensible one given the woman's circumstances.

Through home visiting I learned about the differing attitudes towards all aspects of sexuality of the various ethnic groups and the desperate plight of some unmarried mothers and their children, particularly those of West Indian origin. These continue to need much support from the domiciliary service.

The term 'unwanted' in relation to children took on new meanings. The woman might want a pregnancy to hold on to a man or escape a difficult situation or to feel worthwhile, but might not want a growing child. Women whose own mothering had been deficient had limited capacities for mothering. Their patience and tolerance were soon exhausted, particularly by wilful toddlers. It was (and is) unfortunate that such women may have several children in rapid succession. If their ability to sustain relations was also limited they often had to shoulder the burden of caring for their children alone. I learned that it was both useless and unhelpful to feel angry with such women and the way they treated their children, although this was and is distressing to watch — their own need of good mothering was too great. But they could and did respond to the consistency and reliability of the domiciliary service. Concern, in the face of anger and hostility, directed usually at the vagaries of life, led to trust and from trust grew mutual affection. Many of these women have now through the support of the service successfully persevered with contraception for several years.

As a result of my experience two clear convictions stand out. Firstly, that there has been far too much unnecessary sexual misery. Secondly, that the serious purpose of sex is procreation and that every child has the right to be born wanted and accepted and enjoyed as a unique and precious person. Although a feminist, I believe that every child needs the love and care of *two* parents (whether married or not) and that when a couple decide to have a child, they should only do so when they are prepared to commit themselves to each other for the time taken for the child to grow to emotional maturity and independence.

As members of a caring society and, particularly, as professional 'carers', we should all be concerned that each pregnancy that leads to a child should be the result of an informed, thoughtful and loving decision, as far as is humanly possible.

Introduction

SOCIETAL ATTITUDES TOWARDS SEXUALITY

The last twenty years or so have seen profound changes in society's attitudes towards sex and related matters. Sex, contraception, abortion and venereal diseases are now not only subjects for serious professional study but also for open public discussion, for newspaper and magazine articles and for television and radio. Couples (married and otherwise) now expect to enjoy sex and are presenting themselves for treatment where there are sexual difficulties. Attitudes towards female sexuality, in particular, have significantly altered. Not only is female sexuality given due recognition, but women are now more able to admit that they do not enjoy sex or have orgasms and seek help for this. Premarital sex for both sexes has become more common and with the advent of Gay Liberation in 1970 homosexuality has begun to be seen as a valid expression of a person's sexuality rather than as an illness to be treated. The sexual needs of the handicapped (both physically and mentally handicapped) are beginning to be recognised.

Couples expect to enjoy a sexual relationship free from the fear of unwanted pregnancy. Birth control methods are expected to be safe, convenient and effective. Increasingly, women are wanting not only easy access to abortion but the sole right to determine for themselves whether to have an abortion.

Previously, somewhat Victorian attitudes to sex prevailed. Women were not supposed to be much interested in sex (apart from romance) or to enjoy it. Premarital sex was frowned on for girls, especially, though tolerated for boys (the double standard of morality). Contraception (as well as sex) was not considered an appropriate topic for conversation or public discussion. Indeed, the early family planners such as Bradlaugh, Besant, Marie Stopes and Margaret Sanger drew enormous public calumny upon themselves. Margaret Sanger, in fact, served a short prison sentence for her family planning activities in the United States. An unwanted pregnancy or venereal disease were usually considered the price or punishment for illicit (i.e. pre- or extramarital) sex.

The Kinsey reports (1948, 1953) on the sexual behaviour of over ten thousand American men and women are often credited with initiating the recent change in attitudes, by making the public aware of what people *actually did* rather than what they were supposed by popular folklore to do. (Of course, the earlier influence of other workers such as Freud, Havelock Ellis and Marie Stopes should not be forgotten. Two world wars and the improved status of women also had profound effects on public attitudes towards sexuality.)

During the 1960s a number of additional factors hastened these changes. Among these were increased economic prosperity which led to a healthier population and increased mobility with consequent loosening of family ties, and the 'youth cult'. In Britain, censorship was lifted from books such as *Lady Chatterley's Lover* and the *Kama Sutra* (an Indian sex manual written 1,500 years ago) which deal with sex in an explicit way. The oral contraceptive — the pill — the only method which is practically 100 per cent effective (and reversible) was prescribed, thereby giving women almost complete control over their fertility and allowing them a freedom of choice previously unknown. And in 1967 the abortion law was liberalised.

Around this time anxiety began to be expressed about overpopulation. (It took thousands of years for the world to attain its first billion, the second billion was added in a hundred years and the third in thirty years.) It was increasingly recognised that overpopulation was not solely a Third World problem (England and Wales are the third most densely populated countries in the world, after Bangladesh and Taiwan, with 839 people per square mile).

Premarital sex, particularly among the young, with its resultant casualties — an increase in unwanted pregnancies and venereal disease — began to cause public concern. It was during the 1960s that the increase in teenage pregnancy began to be seen in all Western countries. Increasingly the benefits of successful family planning began to be recognised both for the individual family and for the community as a whole.

In America in 1966 Masters and Johnson (a gynaecologist and psychologist respectively) published their findings after eleven years of work studying the physiology of the human sexual response. They were the first researchers to observe and record the physiological changes that took place during sexual intercourse. Their work has had an important influence on the teaching of sexuality, particularly in American medical schools. The knowledge gained by Masters and Johnson enabled them to derive new techniques for the treatment of sexual difficulties. (The work of Freud, Kinsey and Masters and Johnson will be referred to in greater detail in subsequent chapters.)

PROFESSIONAL ATTITUDES TOWARDS SEXUALITY

The attitudes of the caring professions have tended to lag behind those of the public. Only comparatively few medical students get adequate teaching on sexuality and there is no department of human sexuality in any of our medical schools. It was left to a voluntary organisation, the Family Planning Association, to espouse the cause of family planning in Britain, and it was only in 1974 that family planning became part of the National Health Service.

Social workers, as a professional body, have not been involved in either the development or the delivery of family planning services, in Britain or in the United States. (This has been noted by several authors, including Haselkorn (1968), Allen (1974) and Christopher (1975). The situation is little different with regard to sexual problems (Gochros & Schultz 1972).

Why has there been this reluctance to be involved? One reason must be that there is little programmed teaching on sexuality and contraception on social work courses. It may possibly be mentioned when child care and the family are studied and although teaching may be given on the stages of psychosexual development little is done on practical problems. (The author has led several one-day seminars/workshops in recent years on social work courses where this has been the only teaching given on sexuality.) The corollary of this lack of training is that social workers have failed to define their role in relation to sexual problems and family planning. They have tended to rely on other professionals and have often failed to perceive the barriers that may and do exist to prevent their clients obtaining such help. These comments refer to social workers as a professional group. Obviously individual social workers have seen their clients' needs in these areas and have arranged help for them.

There are of course, more fundamental and contentious issues that may face the social worker in relation to family planning and abortion in particular. These have to do with personal and religious convictions which may prohibit or limit involvement. There are anxieties about seeming to make value judgements and the need to ensure client self-determination. There are also fears that family planning and easy abortion will be seen by society and politicians as the cures for all social ills thereby conveniently ignoring social injustices. These issues will be explored more fully in Parts 2 and 3.

THE PURPOSE AND AIMS OF THE PRESENT WORK

This book is primarily addressed to social work students and community-based social workers. As it is written not by a social worker but by a family planning doctor/psychosexual counsellor working in the grey area between medicine and social work, it would be presumptuous to attempt to teach social work skills. Nor is it intended to turn social workers into sex therapists, family planners or venereologists; rather it is hoped to alert social workers to the needs and difficulties of some of their clients in the area of sexuality and to show how these difficulties can influence (often for the worse) other aspects of the client's life. Further, it is hoped to show that these difficulties, whether experienced in the sexual relationship or in poor fertility control, can profoundly influence the happiness and well-being of the entire family and not just that of the client. Social workers will, it is hoped, be enabled to clarify ways in which to use their special skills, and to define a role for themselves with regard to both sexual and birth control problems. In some cases the social worker may have to work alone; in others there will be a need to refer and/or to work with another agency with more specialist knowledge. It will then be necessary to prepare the client for the experience. It would, therefore, seem essential for the social worker to be reasonably well informed about such matters as the various treatments for sexual difficulties, contraceptive methods, abortion techniques and sexually transmitted diseases.

The book is divided into four parts:

Part 1 — Sexuality   This deals with the theories of psychosexual development, the normal sexual response, a description of the more common sexual difficulties together with the ways in which they present, the influence of class and culture and the different treatment approaches that are available. The sexual needs of the handicapped are considered. Sexual variations, both social and anti-social, are discussed, though the reader is referred to more specialist books for a fuller account.

Part 2 — Family Planning This deals with various aspects of contraception and family planning: the sociology and psychology of family planning, contraceptive methods, attitudes towards them and present-day services. A separate chapter is devoted to groups that need special care with contraception. These are the groups most commonly involved with social service departments.

Part 3 — Abortion This deals with the present law regarding abortion, the diagnosis of pregnancy, abortion techniques, present-day services, the morbidity and mortality of abortion and abortion counselling.

Part 4 — Sexually Transmitted Diseases A description together with the incidence of the more common sexually transmitted diseases (including the venereal diseases) is given. The work of the clinic social worker, especially in relation to contact tracing, is described. Those clients most vulnerable to possible infection are discussed.

Case studies are presented both to illustrate the text and to demonstrate other professional approaches. The majority of the case studies used in the work were in fact shared with social workers (medical, community and residential) in the London Borough of Haringey.

The influence of class and culture on attitudes to sex, contraception, family planning and abortion are also explored, since these vary and must be taken into account when advice or help is offered.

In each Part an attempt is made: (a) to define those clients (or groups of clients) who may be most in need of help or who may be most at risk, e.g. from unwanted pregnancy or sexually transmitted disease, and thus to enable the social worker to identify them; (b) to explore why particular clients (or groups) do have difficulties; (c) to describe the help/treatment available and what the possible role of the social worker might be.

Since several client groups — for example 'the young' — will be found to need special care with all aspects of sexuality, the reasons for this will be dealt with in only one section to avoid repetition.

Finally, there are lists of books and useful addresses.

Note on terminology

Illegitimacy is referred to in various places in the book. The word is used as a convenient form of shorthand. No derogatory or moral stricture is implied or intended. That any child should be labelled legitimate or illegitimate is offensive.

The terms Cypriot, Asian, etc. are used when the influence of culture is examined to refer to groups of people who share a common cultural heritage and do not indicate nationality or citizenship. Many of the young people of those communities have been born in Britain and are British though, obviously, they will be influenced to a greater or lesser extent by their cultural heritage. It may appear to the reader that extreme examples have been used to illustrate cultural attitudes or behaviour but it should *not* be assumed that such patterns of behaviour are manifested by every individual or that the families needing the help of the social services are typical of their respective communities. Nor should it be assumed that Anglo-Saxon culture is homogeneous: this is obviously not so — differences are seen between rural and urban communities, for example. The social worker needs to take this into account and make adjustments when dealing with the particular community with which he is working.

PART 1
Sexuality

1
Sex and the Normal Sexual Response

THE DEVELOPMENT OF SEXUAL IDENTITY

The concern with the role of women, largely brought about by the Women's Movement, has led to the serious study of the possible differences between men and women and of the extent to which these differences (if they exist) are intrinsic, i.e. genetically determined, or artificial and capable of change, i.e. socio-culturally determined. What follows is an attempt to outline the present state of knowledge in an area that arouses much strong emotion which in turn leads to confused thinking.

The foetus in the first six weeks of its life is sexually neutral. After this time, depending on whether it has inherited XY or XX chromosomes, it will develop into a boy (XY) or a girl (XX). The mother always passes on an X chromosome. It is the father who determines the sex of the child by passing on either a Y or an X chromosome through the sperm. The presence of the Y chromosome causes the neutral internal sex organ (gonad) to develop into the testis. Its absence results in the gonad developing into an ovary. The testis then starts to secrete androgens (male hormones). These hormones lead to the development of the male external sex organs. Without androgens the external sex organs develop into female ones. It is postulated (the evidence comes from animal experiments) that the presence of androgens causes the brain to develop differently in the male from the female, thus explaining certain psychological differences.

The sense of maleness or femaleness is established very early on, by about 2½–3 years, and is extremely difficult, if not impossible, to change. Two main theories are put forward to explain the development of sexual identity.

Social Conditioning or Learning Theory Based on their work with children and adolescents of mixed sex anomalies (e.g. pseudohermaphodites — individuals with, say, the male chromosome but with the external sex organs of the female), Money

& Hampson (1957) put forward the idea that a child is sexually neutral at birth but acquires its gender identity and related role behaviour by the way the parents rear it. Thus the mother of a new baby asks first whether it is normal, secondly, whether it is a boy or a girl. The answer determines the parents' attitudes and expectations towards the child, so that they teach it to behave like a boy or a girl (succinctly called the 'blue/pink syndrome'). Thus by a process of learning rather similar to imprinting, the child learns to become a boy or a girl.

Biological Theory According to Hutt (1971), who is highly critical of the social conditioning theory, the most important determining factor is the level of androgens present in the foetus at critical times in its development.

WHAT ARE THE DIFFERENCES BETWEEN THE SEXES?

Biologically, males are more vulnerable to disease and have a shorter life-span than females. Males mature later than females and have greater muscular strength and body size.

Maccoby & Jacklin (1974) in their extensive review of the studies carried out on psychological differences between the sexes feel that the following have been fairly well established:

(1) Girls have, on average, greater verbal ability than boys. This is true of comprehension of difficult written material and verbal fluency.

(2) Boys have, on average, greater visual-spatial and mathematical ability, that is they have greater ability for dealing with visual information and manipulating objects within a spatial context.

(3) Males are more 'aggressive' with sex differences appearing as early as social play does (age 2–3 years). Aggression is defined here as the 'intent of one individual to hurt another, either as such or as part of an attempt to control another for other ends (by use of fear)'. However, the authors also noted that mothers use more physical punishment with boys than with girls, thus possibly setting up a 'circular process where aggression reinforces aggression'. Activity/passivity does not differentiate the sexes unless activity is confused with aggression or activity is regarded as masculine and passivity as feminine, in which case the argument is circular (Seiden 1976).

The following areas were regarded by Maccoby & Jacklin as open to question because of insufficient evidence or ambiguous

findings: sex differences in fear, timidity, anxiety, competitiveness, dominance, compliance, nurturance and 'maternal' (or parenting) behaviour.

Apart from the differences listed above and the fact that the intellectual spread of males is greater than that of females (there are more males than females of very low and very high IQ), most psychological testing has consistently revealed very similar average ability for males and females.

PSYCHOSEXUAL DEVELOPMENT

Prior to Freud's discoveries on infantile sexuality it was believed that children were sexually innocent. If it was discovered that the child was not, then this was blamed on inherited weakness, or 'bad blood', or corruption by an adult. Freud himself originally held the belief that most, if not all, of his female patients had been seduced in childhood by their fathers. He later realised that this was a fantasy held by his patients. Freud believed that there was a force or energy derived from the sexual instinct which needed gratification and was present from birth. This he called the 'libido'. He saw the infant as concerned not only with satisfying its hunger but also with obtaining sexual pleasure. In the first year of life pleasure is derived from sucking and biting (the oral stage). This is followed by the anal stage (1—3 years) when pleasure is obtained from the functions of urinating and defecating. From about 3 to 6 years sensual pleasure is derived from handling the penis in the boy, or clitoris in the girl (the phallic stage). At this time the oedipal phase takes place, in which the child chooses the parent of the opposite sex as the object of his erotic aims and wishes, replacing the parent of the same sex. This arouses both guilt and anxiety, and, in the case of the little boy, fears that his father will punish him for his desires by cutting off his penis (castration fears). The boy's conflicts are resolved by identification with the father and a repression of sexual interest for the next few years (the latent period) until puberty when sexual interest reawakens. Initially the old oedipal conflicts are revived but the task of the adolescent is to detach himself from his parents and find a love object outside the home. In the case of the little girl, the mother is the original love object whom she would like to possess and give a baby to. This being impossible since she lacks a penis (hence penis envy), her sexual longings are focused on father, with

mother as sexual rival. As she fears the loss of mother's love, her secret wishes are suppressed.

Despite the questioning and criticism which Freud's theory of infantile sexuality has faced, many of Freud's claims are objectively true. For example, infantile masturbation and sexual exploration, children's sex play (mothers and fathers, doctors and nurses) and the erotic nature of some aspects of the parent-child relationship are now widely recognised. Later analysts, Erikson (1965) in particular, have extended and developed Freud's theory of psychosexual development by emphasising the psychosocial aspects. What follows is necessarily over-simplified and readers are referred both to Erikson's own account and to that of Skynner (1976) which explores various theories on early development and shows how they relate to each other. According to Erikson, the oral stage is seen as one in which the baby establishes (or fails to establish) basic trust in the parent — of fundamental importance to all subsequent relationships. During the anal stage the first conflict between the needs for personal gratification and social control takes place (the child 'hanging on' to his urine/faeces when the parent wishes him to 'let go' and vice versa). This is the battle for autonomy — the so-called negative phase when the child has to exert his individuality. Too strict parenting at this time may result in a rigid obsessional personality; too lax or inconsistent parenting results in a self-centred personality unable to cope with the give and take required in relationships. The third stage (the phallic or genital) coincides with increasing physical and social independence of the child. The child is intensely curious and needs to explore and test his environment. Erikson saw this as the time when initiative developed. During this stage the child has to learn how to cope with a relationship (that of his parents) rather than relating to one or two people as he did in the two earlier stages.

He has to become aware that he cannot possess the parent of the opposite sex as he would wish but must share him/her, since the parents love each other as well as him. In order for the child to do this successfully, the parents' own sexual relationship must be satisfying and guilt-free so that the child knows he is *not* sexually preferred. He must be in no doubt that the funda-mental loyalty and attraction within the family is between the parents. At the same time the child needs to be aware that a special relationship does also exist between him and the opposite-sex parent. Thus for later sexual happiness the 'little

girl needs to know that her father is a bit in love with her and the little boy that his mother is proud of his masculinity' (Pincus & Dare 1978). The intense feelings between parents and children at this stage would appear necessary for healthy development, provided parents know the boundaries and limitations and do not carry them over to actual sexual experiences as in incest. If the child copes with the pain and jealousy involved in sharing, helped by the love of both parents, he will later be able to cope with the jealousies and exclusions involved in peer group relationships. Thus this stage (according to Skynner, 1976) sees the origins of sharing, of mutuality and reciprocity both in personal sexual relationships and in group interaction. During this time the child becomes increasingly helpful and responsible.

The identification with the same-sex parent which occurs in early childhood is part of the 'working out of the implications of sexual identity' (Skynner 1976). However, this may not be clear-cut since the child may wish to enjoy the advantages of both sex roles and so may adopt the attitudes and interests of the opposite sex as well as those of the same-sex parent. This early modelling upon the parents is later transferred to other admired adults such as teachers and pop stars and also to the peer group. The idea of the sexual self is then tested in relationships with the opposite sex. Finally, the successful completion of psychosexual development is seen in the ability to make and sustain a loving sexual relationship.

The above account presupposes two parents who love each other and their children. There are obviously many ways in which development can go wrong, depending on the quality of parental care and the parental relationship. Much less appears to be known about the effect on psychosexual development of living in a one-parent family, though there will usually be other figures around of the same sex for the child to use as models. However, since the main task to be accomplished during the third stage is learning how to cope with a *relationship* of a couple with all the jealousy and frustration this can entail, it may be that the child reared exclusively in a one-parent household may find sharing in later life, particularly the sharing of a partner with children and vice versa, more difficult.

THE SEXUAL RESPONSE

Although Masters and Johnson's work (1966) conjures up images of white-coated doctors clinically measuring intercourse, this work was essential. Prior to their investigations the medical profession were not only ignorant about the changes that took place but were under serious misapprehensions. For example, it was stated that women lubricated during intercourse as a result of secretions from two glands outside the vagina (Bartholins glands). Masters and Johnson showed that lubrication occurred by means of a 'sweating' reaction through the walls of the vagina. Their work was to have profound consequences for the treatment of sexual problems. This will be examined later.

The physiological responses were observed in approximately 600 men and women ranging in age from 18 to 89 years during more than 10,000 cycles of sexual response. The male and female sexual response were found to have a close similarity. Masters and Johnson divided the male and female sexual response into four successive stages: excitement, plateau, orgasm and resolution. These will be described briefly.

The four stages of the sexual response

1 Excitement phase

Male The penis becomes erect, this being triggered off by stimulation of the penis itself, or by a sexually stimulating sight, or by erotic thoughts. A small penis may double in length. The lengthening of a large penis is less marked. The erection of the penis is due to its engorgement with blood. This is controlled by the involuntary nervous system reflexes which are also influenced by higher brain centres. During love play an erection may be lost and regained several times. When this happens some men fear that they will not regain their lost erection and their anxiety may result in psychological impotence. Men over fifty may find that once they have lost an erection they may not be able to regain it for several hours despite not ejaculating.

Female The first sign of sexual response is the moistening of the vagina, which occurs 10–30 seconds after the initiation of sexual stimulation. The clitoris may become slightly enlarged with blood and may become erect in some women. The size and location of the clitoris bear no relation to a woman's responsive-

ness or her ability to achieve orgasm. Direct contact with the clitoris is not necessary in order to stimulate it. The vagina expands and balloons out; the cervix and uterus are pulled up and back, producing a 'tenting' of the vaginal walls; the vagina increases in length. Women are unaware of these changes, apart from the sensation of becoming wet and feeling sexually aroused. The male is also unaware of these changes apart from the vaginal wetness. These changes were revealed by photographs taken by Masters and Johnson of the internal female organs during sexual activity.

In both sexes the other changes that take place during this stage are: (a) an increase in heart rate and breathing rate, (b) a rise in the blood pressure, and (c) the body muscles become more tense. In the female the nipples become erect and a rash or 'sex flush' spreads over the breasts.

2   Plateau phase

Male   The testes enlarge and are pulled higher into the scrotum. The penis is filled and distended with blood to the limits of its capacity. Two to three drops of fluid may seep from the penis before ejaculation and may contain a few sperm.

Female   The most dramatic change is the appearance of the 'orgasmic platform' from the engorgement and swelling of the tissues surrounding the outer one-third of the vagina. As a result of this swelling the diameter of the lower one-third of the vagina is reduced. It is accompanied by a further ballooning of the inner two thirds of the vagina. The uterus becomes enlarged. The clitoris is elevated from its normal position overhanging the pubic bone and is drawn away from the vagina. The shaft is shortened. The clitoris continues to respond to stimulation, either directly applied or indirectly through the thrusting of the penis into the vagina.

In both sexes the pulse and breathing rate increase, the blood pressure rises further and the muscles become tenser.

3   Orgasmic phase

Male   This is considered the most intensely pleasurable of sexual sensations. Semen spurts out of the erect penis in 3—7 ejaculatory spurts at 0.8 second intervals. The ejaculatory reflex consists of two co-ordinated phases. Firstly, the internal reproductive organs (the vas deferens, the prostate gland, the seminal

vesicles and the internal part of the urethra) contract. The purpose of this is to collect the seminal fluid (i.e. the sperm together with secretions from the seminal vesicles and prostate gland) in the bulbar urethra. Once this has occurred it is very difficult for the man to voluntarily contain his ejaculation. Masters and Johnson have termed the sensations experienced at this stage as those of 'ejaculatory inevitability'. Prior to this stage the man can control the ejaculatory reflex, that is he can prolong intercourse if he wishes. This is in contrast to erection, which is governed by a reflex mechanism which cannot usually be brought under voluntary control. When the ability to control the ejaculatory reflex is lost then premature ejaculation results. The collection of seminal fluid in the bulbar urethra occurs a split second before ejaculation. The second phase of the ejaculatory reflex is *ejaculation* which causes spurts of semen to be forced outward from the penis. This is due to rhythmic contractions of the muscles surrounding the base of the penis, at 0.8 second intervals. This causes the intense pleasure of orgasm. The anal sphincter also contracts. The glans penis is very sensitive after ejaculation.

Female The orgasm is analogous to the ejaculation phase of the male orgasm, though no fluid is discharged. A series of rhythmic contractions of the muscles that form the orgasmic platform in the vagina take place at 0.8 second intervals. In a mild orgasm there may be 3—5 contractions, in an intense one 8—12. The uterus may also contract during orgasm and also the anal sphincter. The male after orgasm is refractory to sexual stimulation for a period of time which grows longer as the male grows older. In contrast, the female, if she wishes, can be stimulated to have further orgasms — the multiple orgasm.

In both sexes the pulse, breathing and blood pressure reach a peak. The face may be contorted into a grimace because the facial muscles tighten. (The woman who says she is experiencing orgasm while looking relaxed and pretty is not being honest!) The muscles of the neck, arms and legs, abdomen and buttocks are also often contracted. There may also be spasm of the muscles of the hands and feet. Men and women may be unaware of these changes at the time though they may ache the next day.

4 Resolution phase

In both sexes the muscular tensions subside and the blood

flows away from the engorged vessels. The heart, breathing rate and blood pressure return to normal within minutes of orgasm.

Male   The penis loses its erection, at first quite quickly though still remaining enlarged, and then much more slowly, over the course of half an hour. In older men the loss of erection takes place more quickly.

Female   It may take half an hour for the female body to return to its unstimulated state. If a woman has not had an orgasm, the resolution may take much longer. The *bodily* responses remain the same whether sexual stimulation is by masturbation, artificial coitus using a vibrator or sexual intercourse. They may occur more quickly when evoked in one way rather than another. For instance it has often been stated that women have slower sexual responses and take a long time to tune up (as if they were rather like a car engine). Women can masturbate to orgasm in seconds. This is perhaps because they know what they like and how they like being touched. It may be that this knowledge is not communicated to the man because in our society men, unlike women, are expected to be experienced and to know what to do. It has been stated that some women can fantasise to orgasm, though none of the women studied by Masters and Johnson showed this. Masters and Johnson also showed that sometimes women just reach the plateau phase and then the sexual excitement dies away. These responses can obtain in the same women at different times. They also found that these physiological changes occurring during sexual activity went on well into old age although at a slower rate.

The work of Masters and Johnson, as mentioned earlier, not only provided accurate information where it had been lacking, but also cleared up some well-known fallacies. For example, it used to be assumed that the circumcised male has less control over ejaculation than the uncircumcised male (the reason being that the circumcised penile glans was more sensitive to external stimuli than the uncircumcised glans). Uncircumcised males were matched at random with circumcised males of similar age. No clinically significant difference could be established between the two. Another widely accepted fallacy was that the larger the penis the more pleasure the woman obtained. The vagina accommodates involuntarily to the penis size, and of greater relevance is the way in which the penis is used. It was also believed that the larger the flaccid penis the larger it becomes

on erection compared to the small flaccid penis. Again, Masters & Johnson (1966 p 191-193) have shown this not to be so. This is not to say that there is not the occasional man with an exceptionally large or small penis.

Another fallacy commonly held, particularly by some women, is about the vagina. They believe that they are 'too small'. The vagina is an elastic 'stretchy' organ and can accommodate a penis of any size. If, however, penetration occurs before the woman is sexually excited, then the woman may complain of pain, tightness and soreness. In those women who have had a large number of children and have lost their muscle tone the vagina may so over-expand during the excitement phases that there is reduced sensation for the man and woman: hence the importance of exercising the vaginal muscles after childbirth. The vagina of a postmenopausal woman may shrink. However, provided that a high level of sexual tension can be achieved, such a vagina will accommodate an erect penis. Hormones can be given by mouth or used locally in the form of cream to counteract the ageing process.

The clitoral versus vaginal orgasm

Until the work of Masters & Johnson it used to be thought that there were two kinds of orgasm in the woman, the clitoral and the vaginal. According to Freud (1905), erotic activity centred on the clitoris in the early stages of psychosexual development. After puberty sexual sensations were transferred from the clitoris to the vagina. The clitoris retained the function of transmitting excitation to the adjacent female sexual parts. Freud used the simile of fine shavings being kindled to set a log of harder wood on fire. Thus the clitoral orgasm was replaced by the vaginal orgasm, and this was thought to constitute psychosexual maturity. Women who obtained their orgasm through stimulation of the clitoris were thought to be immature and phallically orientated and to have failed to come to terms with their feminity. This view has rightly angered feminists, particularly since descriptions of female orgasm have usually been written by men. According to Kaplan (1974), 'The specific controversial question really should be "Does vaginal or clitoral stimulation produce orgasm in women?".' Evidence from Masters & Johnson's work suggests that there is no physiological difference between 'clitoral' and 'vaginal' orgasm. They found no differences in the vaginal reaction — that is the formation of

the orgasmic platform and the rhythmic contraction of the vaginal muscles — in orgasm with sexual intercourse, indirect stimulation of the pubic area or clitoral body stimulation. What may vary is the duration and intensity of the orgasmic experience, which may vary from woman to woman and in the same woman at different times.

Women who achieve orgasm by stimulating the clitoris say it is a sharper, intenser experience than the orgasm achieved through vaginal stimulation alone (Fisher 1973). Clinical experience shows, however, that some women do experience intense pleasure from stimulation of the vagina and cervix. Should such women have a hysterectomy (removal of uterus and cervix) they may complain that sexual sensation and orgasm have changed or been lost.

One possible misunderstanding about the female orgasm is that as women masturbate by rubbing the clitoris (rarely by inserting objects into the vagina) and since the vagina is to all intents and purposes a 'non-existent' organ until the woman has intercourse, which may be in her late teens or twenties, it may take a while for women to become aware of vaginal sensations during intercourse and orgasm.

Ninety per cent of Kinsey's (1953) female informants had experienced orgasm by the age of thirty-five. The stimulus for first orgasm was masturbation for 40 per cent, heterosexual petting for 24 per cent. 17 per cent of the total sample experienced their first orgasm during marital intercourse. However, not all women regularly experience orgasm; Kinsey gives a figure of 42 per cent and Fisher 38 per cent.

How far this is a true picture of female sexuality and how far the result of past negative attitudes to female sexuality remains to be seen.

2
Sexual Difficulties or Dysfunctions

The purpose of this chapter is to describe the various types of sexual difficulties, how they present, their causes and the various treatments available, rather than to turn the social worker into a sex therapist. Nevertheless, as many sexual problems have their origin in ignorance, misinformation and certain types of negative social conditioning received from parents and society, the social worker has a definite role in helping to clear up misunderstandings. Further, as sexual problems are exacerbated by poor communication between sexual partners the social worker can by acting as an intermediary play an important part in overcoming this when sexual difficulties are discussed. This may be all that is required by some couples. Referral for more specialist help may be needed when there is no improvement after using such simple measures. As couples are often anxious about referral, some explanation from the social worker as to what they are to expect will be helpful.

Unfortunately there are not enough facilities and waiting lists tend to be long so that the social worker may have to cope as best he can.

INCIDENCE OF SEXUAL DIFFICULTIES

It is sometimes assumed that sexual difficulties refer to the more exotic sexual variations such as transvestism or exhibitionism. However, the majority of sexual difficulties are to do with unsatisfactory heterosexual intercourse, though it is not possible to give accurate figures. Masters and Johnson estimated that one half of the marriages in the United States are threatened by sexual dysfunctions; one in ten people presenting at a family planning clinic had a sexual problem (Loudon *et al*. 1976).

Sexual difficulties occur in all social classes and cultures. The effect of these will be looked at separately.

TYPES OF SEXUAL DIFFICULTY

Male

Impotence

Impotence, failure to obtain or maintain an erection of the penis, can be either:
  a) *Primary Impotence* The man has not achieved potency in intercourse though he obtains an erection on masturbation
  or
  b) *Secondary Impotence* The man has been able to have erections in the past and to achieve potency in intercourse but is now unable to. This is a common problem. Most men have experienced transient episodes of impotence.
Loss of potency is a devastating experience for a man and it tends to be seen in terms of weakness, loss and death ('Can't get it up', 'It's no use to me').

Premature ejaculation

The man has no control over the ejaculatory reflex. He may ejaculate before penetration of the vagina or after only a few penile thrusts. It can be either:
  a) *Primary* The man has never had control over ejaculation; or
  b) *Secondary* The man has had control in the past.
Primary premature ejaculation is cited in the literature as the most common male sexual disorder. If untreated it can result in secondary impotence. The complaint is 'coming too soon'.

Ejaculatory incompetence

Some men cannot ejaculate intravaginally, though they may ejaculate on manual or oral stimulation by the partner. In more severe cases they can only ejaculate when they masturbate themselves. Masters and Johnson saw only seventeen cases in eleven years and hence thought it was a rare condition. Other workers, e.g. Kaplan (1974), have found the condition more common.

Low sex drive

Lack of interest in sex is commonly due to physical illness, depression, or relationship problems.

Female

The classification of female disorders is not so straightforward as that of the male. It is bedevilled by the word frigidity which has been used as an umbrella-word to refer to a lack of interest in sex and to an inability to achieve orgasm. It is also used as a pejorative word implying that the woman who is frigid is cold and hostile to men. Masters and Johnson advocated the use of 'orgasmic dysfunction' in an attempt to get away from this term and its connotations. Clinical experience shows that whereas women who are not interested in sex rarely obtain an orgasm, those women who complain of lack of orgasm may, nevertheless, be interested in sex and enjoy intercourse.

Lack of interest in sex

a) *Primary* No sexual pleasure has been experienced with any sexual partner.

b) *Secondary* This occurs when women have responded sexually at some time in the past (or with another partner) but the interest is lost. Lack of interest can accompany all the following difficulties.

Non-consummation

Full penetration by the penis into the vagina has not taken place. This can be the grounds for annulment of marriage. Clinically, it is manifested by an intact hymen. Friedman (1962) has described three types of non-consummation:

a) 'The Sleeping Beauty'. This occurs where the woman denies her own sexuality and waits for the man to waken her sexually. Unfortunately, she often chooses a 'safe' partner, i.e. a man who is uncertain of his own sexuality and may suffer impotence. He is often praised as a 'good', nice boyfriend because he did not attempt premarital intercourse.

b) 'Brunhilde'. This refers to the woman who is always looking for a man strong enough to conquer her. She usually chooses as sexual partners men whom she despises.

c) 'Queen Bee'. This refers to the woman who manages to get pregnant without allowing penetration so that she can claim the pregnancy for herself.

Painful intercourse

The woman complains of pain, tightness, smallness or dryness. There may be a physical cause that needs appropriate treatment, or the discomfort can be due to a failure of the woman to get sexually aroused so that the normal sexual responses (enlargement and lubrication of the vagina) do not take place.

Vaginismus

This is a powerful and sometimes painful contraction or spasm of the vaginal muscles. It can be so extreme as to prevent intercourse. The woman may be unaware of the contraction. It is usually discovered on vaginal examination. It may result from past sexual experiences such as rape. However, the main causes are to do with fear, shame and guilt about sex. It may also occur when the woman is angry with the man (e.g. as a result of infidelity) and thus refuses to let him inside her.

Orgasmic dysfunction or lack of orgasm

Primary The woman has never experienced orgasm. She may enjoy love play but does not get beyond the plateau phase of sexual response.

Secondary Orgasm has been experienced in the past. Masters and Johnson sub-divided secondary orgasm dysfunction into three kinds:

a) orgasm with intercourse only;
b) orgasm with masturbation only;
c) occasional orgasm with intercourse which occurs in special circumstances such as on holiday.

In (a) the woman may feel that sexual intercourse is the only permissible form of sexual activity.

In (b) the woman may be able to masturbate herself to orgasm but is unable to have an orgasm with her partner either in intercourse or with his hand stimulating her. In these cases the woman may have fears about 'letting go' and losing control in the presence of another. Yet other women can obtain orgasm with the partner masturbating them but not during intercourse.

Some are satisfied with this and may only present for help when they learn about orgasm during intercourse.

Those women who can only experience orgasm in special circumstances (c) are often extremely inhibited and cannot allow themselves to become sexually excited.

There is an enormous variation in orgasm response, which may explain the difficulty some women have in achieving orgasm during intercourse. At one end of the spectrum are the few women who can fantasise to orgasm without physical stimulation, and at the other, those who need prolonged stimulation either by the penis or by the hand (Kaplan 1974). Only 30% of the women who answered Hite's questionnaire (Hite 1974) reported having orgasm through penile penetration alone.

Lack of orgasm may eventually lead to loss of interest in sex. Although the male and female difficulties have been listed separately they often co-exist; for example, premature ejaculation with primary lack of orgasm, non-consummation with secondary impotence. An untreated problem in one partner can lead to problems in the other.

THE EFFECTS OF AGEING

It has been noted earlier that the sexual response carries on into old age though the changes take place at a slower rate. What may be a normal physiological change may through ignorance or misinformation result in. anxiety that impairs sexual functioning.

For example, the middle-aged man may not be as sexually responsive — that is, obtaining an erection as quickly — as he was in his youth. (Kinsey noted that men are at their sexual peak at eighteen years.) This slower arousal may worry him to such an extent that he becomes impotent, or fears of impotence may lead him into affairs with younger women to prove himself. The older man, in fact, can sustain intercourse longer since the need to ejaculate is not as powerful as in youth.

Similarly, the middle-aged woman may find that she, too, is slower at responding to sexual stimuli. Her anxiety may be such as to prevent normal vaginal lubrication.

Information about these changes may be all that is needed to help such couples.

CAUSES OF SEXUAL DIFFICULTIES

Sexual difficulties are caused by a wide variety of factors. Some are superficial and can easily and quickly be treated in 1—5 sessions, while others are more deep-seated and require much longer treatment, which may not always be successful. In some couples only one partner is affected; in others it is both. However, where a problem persists in one partner the other eventually will be affected. In some cases all the factors will be operating while in others one or two may predominate.

Until recently it was thought that all sexual difficulties had their origins in faulty psychosexual development occurring at a very early age and due to forbidden incestuous fantasies. These largely unconscious fantasies set up a conflict between the wish to enjoy sex and the fear of doing so. This ignores the part played by social and cultural factors together with overt and conscious ways of dealing with sex in the family. The work of Masters & Johnson and the Women's Movement have stressed the significance of socio-cultural factors on sexuality. Kaplan, herself an analyst, supports this (Kaplan 1974) and suggests that 'many other factors besides incestuous wishes can play a role in the genesis of sexual conflicts and dysfunction'. The implications of this view with regard to treatment are profound. If it is assumed that the sexual difficulties are due to unconscious incestuous wishes then analysis would appear to be the only answer. While this may still be necessary for some of the deep-seated sexual problems, many sexual difficulties can be and have been cured by other treatments taking a much shorter time.

Present causes

Ignorance

Despite the plethora of books etc. on sex, many people are still ignorant about their bodies, their sex organs and how they function. The clitoris in particular seems a mysterious organ. Couples often present saying they cannot find it. Ignorance is invariably accompanied by poor sexual technique. There may be false expectations of the sex act and the performance required of the sexes. A common fallacy is that only large penises can give women orgasms. Thus if his partner does not get an orgasm the man may believe his penis is too small. Simultaneous orgasm without the use of hands is regarded as the epitome of the perfect sex act (a notion encouraged by certain romantic novelists).

Fear

There may be a fear of sex — fear of its power, fear of being overwhelmed or changed by it, fear of losing control and being thought weak. Joyful sex means abandonment, losing oneself, an experience too threatening for the person who needs to be 'in charge'. For some women abandonment is synonymous with depravity and must be guarded against. There is a fear of pain, fear of being damaged or of damaging and a fear of the sex organs themselves. Women fear being ripped and torn, men fear hurting women or having their penises damaged by the vagina. There is a fear of failure and of being found 'lacking'.

Anxiety

This is allied to fear and accompanies many sexual problems. On a physiological level anxiety and fear exacerbate sexual problems, either by preventing sexual arousal (and thereby directing blood that should go to the pelvic organs, to enlarge the penis and vagina, to go instead to the muscles) or switching excitement off once it has occurred. Masters and Johnson gave a special term, 'performance anxiety', to the situation where a man who has previously failed to obtain or sustain an erection watches himself anxiously on each sexual occasion to see whether it will occur again. Unfortunately, his anxiety ensures that erection will not take place, for reasons mentioned above.

Embarrassment, shame and guilt

These feelings are commonly associated with sex, especially where it is believed that the 'good' person is really asexual. Considerable guilt may be experienced over sexual fantasies, particularly those associated with masturbation. These feelings may be so intense as to prohibit even talking about sex either with the partner or with a professional person. Deep disgust with sex may militate against successful treatment. This disgust often manifests itself in an over-concern with personal hygiene which can be obsessive, with a dislike of vaginal secretions and semen. Sex is equated with 'mess', 'dirt' and 'excreta'.

The causes listed so far tend to go together. At the superficial level they can easily be treated with straightforward re-education, helping the person to feel that his or her sexuality is acceptable. At a deeper level these feelings and even ignorance itself may be due to a strong need to repress and deny sexuality, either to guard against incestuous fantasies or to preserve an image of the self as an asexual and therefore 'good' person. Long-term treatment may then be necessary to alter this.

Failure to communicate and unrealistic expectations

Many couples with sexual difficulties have never discussed sex together or their own feelings, needs, desires. This can result from embarrassment or fear. It is feared that if they say what they like, this may be interpreted as criticism or rejection. Certain societal attitudes reinforce these feelings, namely, that men are expected to 'know' what to do (since they are experienced) while women are sexually innocent. Consequently, some men do feel threatened if their partner attempts to suggest what to do. Some women collude over this and pretend that they do enjoy sex or have orgasms. Should they present for treatment because they do not enjoy sex or have orgasms, they may insist that their partner must not be involved in treatment, to avoid having to admit deceit. This may be accompanied by fears of damaging male ego and thus producing impotence. 'I don't want to hurt him', 'I don't think he could take it' are common remarks in this context. Unrealistic expectations of the partner or of sex nourished by ignorance may lead to disappointment, which in time may cause resentment and hostility. This again prevents communication. Some women expect their partner to give them orgasms, without any involvement on their part. Allied to this is a fantasy that somewhere there is a 'perfect' lover who will do the right things. Some men feel they should be in charge and be responsible for the women's orgasm. Underlying this may be an anxiety about potency or penis size. When a sexual problem does arise the couple may not be able to discuss it openly but rather may accuse each other of not caring or being unfaithful. Some couples are unable to share their feelings on any topic, not just sex. They are unable to 'let go' in any sense — get really angry, for example. Feelings, or rather the expression of them, is thought to be dangerous and destructive.

Collusive patterns in relationships

Certain sexual difficulties seem to go together and reflect the collusive adjustment which some couples make early on in their relationship. Only when one of the partners wishes to change (for whatever reason) will the difficulty of the other be unmasked. Thus the woman who is afraid of sex and her own sexuality may choose a sexually 'safe' man, that is, one who makes few sexual demands. During courtship they often compliment themselves on finding a really 'nice' (asexual) person — someone whom they can safely introduce to parents. After marriage the woman may feel it is all right to be sexual, whereupon she finds that her partner is not much concerned. She may then present with a complaint of losing her interest in sex. Men whose masculine image and potency depend on the belief that women are inferior tend to marry 'little girl' wives uncertain of their own sexuality. Sex may be satisfactory for a time. Should the little girl grow up, the man may become impotent.

Past causes

Children are not born with sexual difficulties (unless these relate to a physical disability) nor are they born guilty, anxious, and fearful about sex. They learn to become so. 'Learning about sex in our society is learning about guilt' (Gagnon & Simon 1973). This is the legacy of Judaeo-Christian teaching about sex. Emphasis was given to reproductive sex by Judaism; other forms of sexual expression — oral sex, masturbation, homosexuality — were considered abnormal since they did not lead to reproduction. Christianity, under the influence of St Paul and later St Jerome, stressed the importance of celibacy which was considered a superior state (that is, closer to God) than the sexual one. St Paul did, however, advise that it was better 'to marry than to burn' with sexual desire. Later, when the cult of the Virgin Mary took hold, the perfect idealised woman was the asexual mother. (For the evolution of the cult from the romantic love concepts of the French troubadours of the eleventh century, see Warner 1976.) As a result of these influences, arising partly as a reaction to Graeco-Roman hedonism, sexuality took on its essentially negative connotations. Female sexuality suffered particularly. The good woman was asexual. It followed from this that the woman who showed any interest in sex or had sexual feelings was bad. Thus the concept of two kinds of women took shape. This reached its extreme manifestation in Victorian society, from whose attitudes we are emerging (Seymour Smith 1975, Wayland Young 1965). Inevitably parents imbued with society's attitudes passed these on to their children who grew up either knowing very little about sex or believing it to be wrong, depraved or dirty. Although sex is now more freely discussed, there are still many families in which it is never mentioned, or, if it is, is accompanied by dire warnings. Thus many people in our society learn nothing positive and good about sex and do not receive parental permission to be sexual. The child will find difficulty in accepting his sexuality when the parents are not proud of theirs. The mother who despises herself for 'feminine weakness' or feels that her genital organs make her vulnerable conveys this to her daughter, who may reject her own sex organs. Sometimes the person believes that they have no right to sexual pleasure denied to the parents. Paradoxically, perhaps, sex can only be enjoyed when it can be considered sinful. Thus some women enjoy sex before marriage (rebelling against parents) but not afterwards when sex is permissible.

The kind of family in which the child grows up can affect later sexual behaviour. Thus the couples mentioned earlier who are afraid to show their feelings have usually been reared in families where feelings were suppressed or denied. Children deprived of parental love often need physical proof of love and may, in consequence, make excessive sexual demands to reassure themselves. Failure to comply leads to accusations of unfaithfulness. Children reared in a predominantly one-sex household may have difficulty in relating to the opposite sex and nourish fears and fantasies about them. The boy reared in a household of women, particularly if they are demanding and hard to please, may later experience problems with potency since he may feel he can never satisfy women. Unresolved feelings of anger, disappointment, envy or fear of the opposite-sex parent may be carried over into a sexual relationship so that attempts are made to thwart the partner's sexuality. For example, the woman reared in a family where boys were preferred, especially by the father, may be envious of men and may not allow them to be potent with her. The child who is made a favourite by one parent, because of an unsatisfactory marriage, may experience later ambivalence about his sexuality. There may be a reluctance to give up the position of 'dad's girl' or 'mum's boy', especially where the child is made to feel guilty about loving someone else. A failure to develop sexual confidence can occur where a sibling is more physically attractive and comparisons are constantly made.

Looking at particular sexual difficulties: *potency* in the man is intimately bound up with what he feels about himself — his effectiveness and confidence as a man. The impotent man tends to believe that it is only his penis which is 'weak', whereas exploration of other areas of his life reveals impotence, too. Primary *premature ejaculation* results from a failure to control sexual excitement, as a result of anxiety. It occurs with a sexual partner and not with masturbation. Young men tend to be easily excited sexually and ejaculate quickly. This behaviour is reinforced by sexual encounters where speed is at a premium, e.g. for fear of being caught. This may then later persist in marriage where it may be taken for the norm until the woman complains of being unsatisfied. Help may then be sought. Men with *ejaculatory incompetence* are usually fearful of parenthood and/or fear a rival (the child) for the woman's affection. Sexual problems in the female tend to be more the result of a denial both of sexuality itself and of themselves as sexual people.

Causes of secondary sexual difficulties

As has already been noted, some sexual difficulties may lead to others, e.g. premature ejaculation may eventually lead to secondary impotence or a problem in one partner can lead to one in the other. Other causes of secondary sexual difficulties have to do with an altered life situation — stress of any kind, financial and domestic worries, fear of pregnancy, a difficult childbirth, guilt over an abortion, physical and mental ill health, fatigue, premature ageing, drugs used to treat illness, drug addiction, alcoholism, relationship or marriage breaking up, unfaithful partner, guilt over a secret affair. Alcoholism has a particularly devastating effect on male sexuality, causing secondary impotence though sexual desire may still be present. Sexual boredom may occur in couples who have previously had a satisfactory sexual life, possibly as a result of predictability. Fantasies about the supposed exciting sex life of others can cause unnecessary dissatisfaction and difficulties. Sometimes one partner insisting on making love in a particular way or wanting the other to do something the other finds distasteful can result in sexual difficulties. For example, the man may want oral sex which the partner finds distasteful; if he persists in his demands, the woman may eventually be totally unresponsive sexually.

PRESENTATION OF SEXUAL DIFFICULTIES

Direct complaint

This is occurring with increasing frequency as societal attitudes towards sex become more open. However, the fact that people do nowadays feel more able to state that they have sexual difficulties may divert the social worker from looking at other problems which the individual (or couple) has but which are too painful to reveal. For example, a recently married woman complained of painful intercourse which she thought was due to a minor gynaecological operation. Examination revealed nothing abnormal. It took several interviews before the woman could admit that she was disappointed in her marriage and resented her husband's childlike dependence on her.

Complaint about the partner

The man or woman may present with complaints about the partner's inadequacy or problem. These should not be accepted at face value. They may well hide fears and anxieties about the self. For example, the man who complains that his partner's vagina is too large or that he does not get enough sensation may worry that his penis is too small. The woman who says 'All men are like that, just after one thing' may be referring to a brutish husband but she may equally be refusing to acknowledge or accept her own sexuality. The woman who says 'He can't get enough' with excitement in her voice may be needing reassurance about her own sexual desires. Some men and women present themselves and their difficulties in a seemingly altruistic manner that can be very deceptive to the unwary. They usually present as being only there for the partner, saying they would not come for themselves as they are not really bothered. Behind this altruism may lie deep resentment and disappointment with the partner. Thus a man may present himself as kind and thoughtful, he does not want to hurt his wife. Underlying this may be anger and hostility with his wife for her lack of response. Or a woman may say it does not mean anything to her but she has come for his sake. In reality she may be asking for him to be changed into the good lover for whom she had 'saved' herself.

Sexual difficulties can also present indirectly or disguised as other problems. The following are some of the ways in which they can present.

Contraceptive problem

There may be conflict over the method used, which partner uses a method or a conflict over whether contraception is used at all. Sometimes these conflicts are to do with envy and resentment of the partner's sexuality and a wish to control or limit it by not using contraception. This particularly refers to certain women who find sex distasteful or disgusting. Where sex is regarded as solely for procreation and not for pleasure the woman may have great difficulty in choosing and/or persevering with a method. No method is considered suitable. There are frequent complaints about the methods. The woman or man may only allow themselves to become sexually excited when there is a risk of pregnancy. This can lead to 'contraceptive roulette'. Methods may be scapegoated for loss of interest in sex. (This is explored more fully in Part 2.)

A sexual problem may manifest itself when a woman is being examined vaginally, though she may have been unable to admit that she has a problem. Spasm of the vaginal muscles and a reluctance to be examined, which can be so extreme that the thighs are held tightly together, usually indicates that the woman is afraid and anxious about intercourse. The vaginal examination can reveal much about the woman's attitudes to sex, her own body and sexuality. (This will be dealt with in more detail in the section on treatment, pp. 55–56.)

Infertility problems

The couple may present when they have failed to conceive, or they may want to adopt a child. It is only on tactful and sensitive enquiry that a sexual problem is revealed. Non-consummation, impotence, premature ejaculation and ejaculatory incompetence can all present as an infertility problem. The knowledge that the couple or one of the partners is infertile can lead to sexual difficulties such as a loss of interest in sex.

Medical and gynaecological problems

Sexual problems can present under the guise of tiredness, head-aches, stomach-aches and backaches for which no physical cause can be found. Complaints by women of vaginal discharges and irregular or prolonged periods can also indicate sexual difficulties. Venerophobia or repeated induced abortions may cover up a sexual problem. The person may feel so guilty and ashamed of his sexual desires that he feels he needs to be punished by getting venereal disease. Repeat abortions may similarly be used as self-punishment for having sexual desires and sexual relationships.

After hysterectomy a woman may no longer believe she is sexually attractive and since she cannot get pregnant cannot allow sex just for pleasure. She may not be able to admit this and instead presents with tiredness and depression.

Relationship, marital and family problems

Sexual difficulty can present as a relationship, marital or family problem. It can be difficult to work out which came first; often they co-exist. For some couples sex is the only part that is satisfactory and in yet others the relationship is good but the sex is bad. But for many couples a sexual difficulty eventually affects the relationship or marriage and vice versa. Arguments about money and possessions often have a sexual problem as their basis: she refuses sex, he is mean with money. Struggles for control and dominance within the relationship or marriage often get reflected in the sexual relationship. Thus if the woman fears male domination she may never give herself completely during intercourse and cannot allow herself to have an orgasm since this would indicate that she was weak and had lost control. The man who wants to show how 'strong' he is may insist on taking the sexual initiative on all occasions.

Problems associated with childbirth

Sexual problems frequently present after a new birth, particularly the first. Some mothers, believing that the task of sex is now accomplished lose interest in it and take on a 'Madonna' image, i.e. mothers cannot be lovers. Much of this feeling is a carry-over from childhood feelings that their own mothers were asexual beings. In new mothers there tends to be an emotional absorption with the baby which can make the husband feel excluded. There is the physical reality of tiredness, broken nights and emotional demands of a baby that may well make the woman uninterested in sex. If the husband is immature and needs his wife as a mother also, he may begin to make impossible demands upon her, both sexually and otherwise, which lead to resentment. Extramarital affairs may take place at this time. A painful delivery can also lead to non-interest in sex in the woman and fear on the part of the man about damaging his wife and/or damaging his penis. Breast feeding can also pose problems. The breasts form an important erotic zone. The husband may be jealous that these now 'belong' to the baby, even if only temporarily. The birth of a handicapped child can also lead to sexual difficulties. The woman, in particular, is often horrified that her body could have produced such a child.

Children's problems presented to the social worker or child guidance clinic may prove to be a manifestation of the parents' sexual and marital difficulties. A young mother complained to her health visitor about her baby. He was always crying and she feared what she might do to him. The baby was physically healthy and the mother was referred to the social services. The social worker did a domiciliary visit and an all-too-familiar but sad picture emerged. The young couple had courted in their teens, she had to get married because she became pregnant. She had never enjoyed sex much but was flattered that someone 'fancied her'. She had had a difficult pregnancy and had used this as an excuse to refuse intercourse. After the baby's birth the husband not unnaturally hoped all would be well. However, the wife was always tired as a result of sleepless nights with the baby. She was not interested in sex. The husband, fed up with repeated rebuffs, had started to go out drinking. She (and he) began to blame the baby for all their troubles. The husband and wife knew very little about sex and about their bodies and were unable to discuss their sexual feelings with each other. The husband was anxious about the size of his penis and was convinced that his wife did not enjoy sex because he was not big enough; when asked why he thought that, he replied that his mates had always teased him, telling him that he must have a small one since he was a small man. In his anxiety about himself he had also convinced himself that as he was not 'getting it' from his wife another man must be, which was another source of quarrels between them.

Adolescents with their growing sexual attractiveness and energy can also place a strain on the parents' sexual and marital relationship, particularly as their development tends to occur at a time when the parents are losing their youth and sexual attractiveness. This can result in much family tension and jealousy.

CLASS & CULTURAL ATTITUDES TO SEX

The preconceived ideas and myths that we all have about people from other social classes and cultures determine our view of their problems and of solutions to them that may be quite inappropriate. Thus the professional helper has to be aware not only of the different attitudes, but also of his own to see how far they influence his views of the situation. For example, professional people who are often middle-class often believe that the working class are 'randier' and 'always at it' and are freer from the restraints and inhibitions of the middle class. There is no evidence so far available to support this view. Kinsey's findings mentioned earlier showed that working-class women in particular are far less likely to enjoy sex and are more inhibited than other groups. Rainwater (1960, 1964, 1965) confirmed these findings, though on a smaller sample. Cultural differences with regard to sex have not been examined in such depth as class differences, apart from those done on pre-literate, primitive peoples (Mead 1929, Malinowski 1927, Murdoch 1949).

The descriptions of the attitudes given below are obviously generalisations, and not all people belonging to a particular class or culture will share or manifest all its attitudes towards sex, particularly with the growth of the feminist movement and the expectations of individuals that sex should be pleasurable for them.

Class attitudes

Working-class attitudes

Parents find it very difficult to discuss sex with their children. There is a very real problem of language since usually only the 'dirty' words (Anglo-Saxon) are used rather than the polite medical ones (usually Latin). This makes discussion about sex virtually impossible because the words available are rude or swear words. There are strong taboos against masturbation and children found touching their sexual organs are told to 'stop it or I'll cut it off' if they are boys, or 'stop fiddling with yourself' if they are girls. Working-class boys grow up with the attitude that they should stop masturbation as early as they can and substitute heterosexual activity; hence they tend to begin intercourse earlier than middle-class boys (noted by Kinsey *et al*. 1948, Schofield 1965). For working-class girls masturbation is usually not even considered since it is thought to be a perversion. The double standard of morality operates, so that boys are expected to be experienced and to know all about sex, while a 'good' girl is hard to persuade to have sex but a 'bad' one is easy and then gets a reputation. Since the man is expected to know all about sex there is enormous anxiety about losing face and admitting ignorance. Women (and wives) collude with this. They may present at a clinic or surgery saying that they do not enjoy sex and take the blame on themselves. They very often do not want either to discuss sex with their partners or involve them in treatment. Usually they have pretended to their partners that sex was enjoyable and so to try to discuss this with them would be to admit their pretence and deceit. This can prove difficult to treat, especially since an integral part of treatment consists of trying to get couples to share their feelings and needs. Ignorance about the position and function of the clitoris is commonly found. Sex magazines have been an enormous help here. Different sexual positions, sex with the light on, sex other than at night and oral sex are usually frowned on (though the men want 'to experiment') from the belief that any position other than the 'missionary' (male superior) one is perverse. Realistically, of course, many working-class homes are overcrowded and lack privacy so that the sex magazines' advice to strip off and have sex in the living room whenever you feel like it is a non-starter. Another problem is the sharing of homes with in-laws, with the constant anxiety that mother or mother-in-law will barge in. This is where simple advice like putting a lock on the bedroom door may be all that is needed. However, that too can make women self-conscious and may account for that group of women noted, by Masters & Johnson, to have only occasional orgasm, for example when they are away on holiday. Another prevalent working-class view is that at a certain age you are, or should be, 'past it'. Women who have seen sex as another household chore heave a sigh of relief at the menopause since they can use it as an excuse not to have sex.

Yet another common finding is that sex, especially for the woman, is really for 'making babies' and certainly not for personal pleasure. There is usually associated distaste with the sexual organs and a positive aversion to touching them (hence problems with the mechanical methods of birth control to be dealt with later).

Of course, attitudes are changing so that women, particularly, will ask questions like 'Will the pill help me to enjoy it?', 'Why don't I enjoy it?', or 'I've read this book about women and it mentions something called the clit... I can't pronounce it — what is it?'

Middle-class attitudes

It is perhaps among the middle class that attitudes have changed most markedly. Middle-class parents, especially the younger generation, are more likely to talk about sex to their children. Words are less of an embarrassment since they know the 'proper' i.e. medical, words. They are less likely to admonish their children if they catch them masturbating. Middle-class young people are more likely to continue masturbating till later ages and have intercourse later than working-class young people (Kinsey *et al.* 1948, 1953, Schofield 1965, Farrell 1978). When middle-class girls do start having intercourse, they are more likely to attend a clinic for birth control advice. The double standard of morality seems to have less of a hold in the middle class. Women's sexuality, particularly influenced by the Women's Movement, is more accepted. Their sexual needs and desires are more likely to be recognised. Middle-class couples tend to talk more openly to each other about sex and are more likely to present sexual difficulties together as a couple. Middle-class women, being more widely read, are better informed and know more about their bodies and sex organs than working-class women. There is less reluctance in examining their own bodies and a greater acceptance of birth control methods such as the cap that require the woman to examine her vagina. Experimenting with different sexual positions and oral sex also seems to be more acceptable. However, the sexual expectations among the middle class, influenced by the growing body of information about sex, may be unrealistically high, with demands for a perfect sexual performance and multiple orgasms every time. This in itself is the cause of some sexual difficulties among young middle-class couples.

All this is in direct contrast to the Victorian attitudes that prevailed, though modified, among the middle class until fairly recently. In Victorian times, of course, female sexuality, particularly that of middle-class women, was negated. Thus a practising physician could remark in the 1850s, 'I should say that the majority of women (happily for society) are not much troubled with sexual feeling of any kind' (Acton 1857).

Working-class couples may experience more difficulty in verbalising their feelings and needs. Part of the treatment may have to concentrate on this to enable the couple to express and share their feelings, good and bad.

Middle-class couples, on the other hand, though more used to discussing their feelings may use words as a defensive barrier. They may 'intellectualise' their difficulties and while seeming to be insightful may effectively deny the therapist's interpretations and refuse to really share their feelings with each other.

Cultural attitudes

A description of some of the different cultures to be found in Britain is given in Chapter 14, particularly with respect to marriage customs and attitudes to family size and fertility control. At the risk of oversimplification, only sexual attitudes will be examined here, though it must be stressed that these tend to be intimately bound up with those towards marriage and procreation. It also needs to be stated that adherence to cultural norms depends heavily on education level and religious conformity: those who are less well educated and more conformist are more likely to maintain cultural norms.

However, many individuals may well be in a transitional stage between their culture of origin and that of Britain. This may lead to intergenerational conflict between those (usually the old) who wish to preserve their culture and those (usually the young) who wish to abandon it or at least some aspects of it. This is particularly relevant to those practices relating to sex, marriage and the family.

Asian and Cypriot

These communities tend to be male-dominated and patriarchal, and despite religious differences (Indian — Hindu, Pakistani, Bangladeshi; Turkish Cypriot — Moslem; Greek Cypriot — Orthodox Christian), show many similar attitudes to sexuality,

particularly female sexuality. Sex education is almost totally
lacking except that relating to personal hygiene and the need
for modesty, especially for girls. Among Moslems the genital
organs are accorded special respect and children are taught from
an early age to clean themselves carefully after urinating and
defecation. Masturbation is frowned upon and homosexuality
is regarded as abnormal. The double standard of morality tends
to operate so that although premarital sex may be condoned or
at least tolerated for boys, it is strictly forbidden for girls.
Indeed, sex education for girls is centred on the need for a girl
to be a virgin when she marries. This led in Hindu and Moslem
society to child marriage. The girl was married off soon after
puberty (usually to a much older man), since it was believed
that the longer she remained unmarried the greater the risk of
her losing her virginity. Thus girls before marriage are closely
chaperoned. Marriages are arranged and are more in the nature
of a business transaction than a love match. Sex is regarded as a
duty which must result in children, particularly sons. For
Hindus sex is a sacred duty and part of religious observance.
Little regard is paid to female sexuality among these communities. Women are not supposed to be interested in sex and are
there to satisfy the needs of their husbands. Moslem men are
told to regard women as their fields and to till them whenever
they wish. Not surprisingly, perhaps, problems relating to sex
are usually to do with the inability to conceive or proof of
virginity. For the man to admit a sexual problem such as impotence or premature ejaculation means an extreme loss of face,
and the woman may be blamed for any problem. (A Cypriot
man, rather than admit his impotence, proclaimed that his new
wife was not a virgin. Since the consequences of this were
extremely serious for the woman, her family took her to a
gynaecologist who found that she was definitely a virgin. Once
challenged, the man continued for a time to accuse his wife, but
eventually admitted his problem.) The man may present alone
with his sexual difficulty but refuse to involve his wife. There
are usually extreme anxieties about secrecy and the need to
keep both families in ignorance. The man might have been
potent with prostitutes before marriage but impotent with his
wife, who may be regarded as too 'pure' for sex. Language may
be more of a barrier for women than for men, and women
(apart from the more educated) rarely present with sexual
difficulties, especially with those which relate to their own
needs such as a lack of interest in sex or lack of orgasm. Rather

they may present (brought by their husbands) with non-consummation or painful intercourse, particularly where there is anxiety about conceiving. In these cultures the family is all-important. Little attention is paid to the needs or desires of individuals and thus there is little discussion about feelings. Allied to this is resignation and acceptance of one's fate. Thus when a sexual problem is presented there may be extreme reluctance to discuss feelings and a failure to see their relevance. Help is seen in terms of drugs or operations. Here directive therapies — telling couples what to do — may be more useful than counselling.

Irish

The influence of the Catholic Church is paramount. Both sexes are reared modestly and told very little about sex, except for being warned about the evil consequences. Girls attending convents are forbidden to show their bodies to other girls. Both boys and girls must guard against sinful, i.e. sexual, thoughts and self-abuse (masturbation), and to confess both if they occur. Both sexes tend to be embarrassed by sex. Since men are not expected to be experienced they are usually as ignorant as the woman. Non-consummation is a not uncommon problem. Women are usually the ones who present the sexual problem. There may be complaints of painful intercourse, lack of interest and dryness. This is related to the fact that they cannot allow themselves to get sexually excited. Sexual difficulties are often discovered by chance on vaginal examination when spasm of the vaginal muscles is found. Since sex is seen primarily for procreation, there may be conflicts over contraception and refusal of sex after hysterectomy or the menopause. Couples can have great difficulty in discussing sex together, owing to extreme shyness and embarrassment. Oral sex or sexual positions other than the male superior position are often unacceptable. Women are usually ignorant about their bodies. This may be accompanied by profound disgust with the sex organs which may be impossible to overcome. Treatment needs to emphasise re-education and talking about sex in a relaxed way. The therapist's role needs to be that of a good parent who can sanction sexual activity and provide acceptance of the sexual self.

West Indian

Sexual activity and sexual pleasure for both sexes seem much more acceptable in West Indian culture, despite little or no formal sex education within the home. The double standard of morality is not in evidence. Premarital sex is acceptable and illegitimacy is not a social stigma for historical reasons.

Both masturbation and homosexuality are regarded as abnormal. Adolescent West Indian boys tend not to masturbate or to be reluctant to admit that they do. Clinical experience in Haringey suggests that sexual intercourse seems to take place earlier among West Indian young people (early or mid-teens) than others. This may also obviate the need to masturbate. Women accept their sexual organs and expect to enjoy sex. There is a mistaken belief that women discharge, i.e. ejaculate on orgasm, like men. Sex is likely to be discussed openly between couples with little embarrassment. Women tend to be more directly critical of their partners: 'He's no good to me', meaning their partner is impotent. Men are anxious lest they do not please their women sexually. Failure to do so or the woman leaving for another man is likely to precipitate premature ejaculation or problems with potency in the man. Once a sex problem does occur it can be difficult for the individual or couple to accept that there is not a physical cause since sex is seen as a natural function. Thus it is usually expected that drugs will be given for treatment. Directive approaches rather than counselling may be more appropriate.

TYPES OF TREATMENT FOR HETEROSEXUAL DIFFICULTIES

The treatment will be covered from an historical point of view since this may demonstrate the limitations of the older types of therapy and the necessity for new approaches. Therapy for sexual problems is at present in a state of flux in Britain. Evaluations of the different kinds of treatment have not yet been carried out. At the moment Masters & Johnson therapy, or a modified form of it, is in vogue. Its limitations may only be discovered after more widespread use. Since sexual dysfunctions may have a variety of causes, some superficial, others more deep-seated, successful treatment may well depend on an eclectic approach rather than a didactic one (Wright *et al*. 1977).

Psychotherapeutic/psychoanalytic approach

It is possible that sexual problems were largely ignored because of the powerful influence of Freudian theory and the feeling that only long-term analysis, which is expensive and time-consuming, would cure the difficulties. Until the 1950s this was the only form of treatment available. For certain sexual problems the psychoanalytic approach may be the best one, particularly where the guilt about incestuous fantasies is strong. Success will lie in the correct selection of cases for this form of treatment.

Brief psychotherapy/psychosexual counselling : the Balint Approach

Sexual problems were and are often presented at family planning clinics, either consciously stated ('Sex hurts', 'I don't enjoy sex', and so on) or unconsciously revealed by ambivalence over contraception and anxiety and fear of the vaginal examination. Doctors working in this area were conscious of their lack of expertise although individual doctors such as Joan Malleson and Helena Wright had attempted to treat sexual problems and, indeed, had written books describing their work as guides for other doctors.

In the late 1950s a group of family planning doctors approached Michael Balint (then working as an analyst at the Tavistock Clinic) with a view to devising a training scheme along the lines that Balint was then using to train general practitioners. Balint helped to start the seminar-training technique for family planning doctors in which a group of eight doctors meet fortnightly under the leadership of a trained doctor or psychoanalyst over a period of time (usually 2—4 years). Cases are presented and the doctors' attitudes and approach, and the doctor/patient relationship, are explored. Balint taught GPs that they could use the 'doctor' as medicine. In the same way family planning doctors undergoing this training were taught how to explore feelings and to use the feelings engendered in them by the patients and reflect these back to them. This is novel for both patients and doctors. Patients when seeing a doctor usually expect to be given drugs and indeed when they present with sexual problems often ask for tablets or hormones to help them to avoid the pain of looking at their own and their partner's feelings. Doctors, of course, often collude. Their training has usually focused on drugs and operations (that is, the doctor *does* something) as treatment. Thus men complaining of impotence to their GP may well be given hormones though there is no evidence that their benefits are other than short-term except for a small minority of men. A placebo could well suffice in their place.

Treatment is focused on the presenting person, rather than the couple. Sending for the partner is considered to be a reflection of failure on the part of the doctor to adequately come to grips with the problem. It may also direct attention from the presenting person and may be a collusive acceptance with the patient that it is the partner's fault. It is perhaps no wonder that if and when the partner does come he/she is usually angry and in no mood to be treated. Oedipal conflicts are not dealt with in depth and the aim is to treat in 5—10 sessions. An extensive formal sexual history is not taken since it will be revealed by the patient himself as he presents and discusses his difficulty. Use is made of the present — the here and now of the situation. For example, how did the patient come to be referred (was the referrer made to feel hopeless and impotent by the patient?) and what hopes and expectations of treatment does he bring? Is the doctor seen as all wise and all powerful — the parent who will make everything better? Or is the doctor being set up in order to be knocked down so that the patient can say 'Look I've tried everything — no one can help me' and use this as a weapon over the partner? Clues to feelings and attitudes are provided by the patients, how they enter the room, how they are dressed, their manner, the way they sit and so on. The young woman who is dowdily dressed and sits with drooping head proclaims loudly that she does not think much of her sexual attractiveness or sexuality. Failure to recognise and comment on these aspects can prolong treatment unnecessarily. Much of human communication (and certainly between couples) is by non-verbal means. Recognition of and comment on the signals put out makes the person feel that they really are understood and that due respect is being paid to their dignity and worth. A doctor's question asked in a cheery manner, 'And how are you today?', completely ignored a woman's depressed demeanour which the doctor had registered mentally but failed to comment on. The doctor was surprised that the woman failed to keep subsequent appointments.

Social convention often required that hostility and anger be either glossed over or responded to in kind, thereby missing the possible underlying anxiety or the reason for the anger. An angry man presented at a clinic saying his wife was frigid and that someone had better do something or he would leave her. The doctor noted the anger and remarked 'You seem very cross — it must be upsetting and hurtful that your wife does not respond to you.' The acknowledgement of his anger and possible pain enabled him to admit that he was worried about his own potency. The person who is anxious to please may actually be nurturing a great deal of unexpressed anger. The person who is very nice and never loses his temper may actually be afraid to do so and may fear the loss of love as a consequence. The doctor can allow the expression of these painful and uncomfortable feelings and can, by still showing that he cares, show that these feelings will not destroy the person. The patient may make the doctor feel depressed or angry or frustrated or impotent. This is used in interpretation. For example, the woman who complains of a lack of interest in sex and seems to expect the doctor to do all the work, urging him on to further heights of endeavour, may well be doing this to her partner, who understandably gets fed up with the situation. The doctor has to bring this out into the open and say: 'You seem to expect me to do all the work without giving very much yourself. This makes me feel pretty frustrated as if I never can do enough to please you. I wonder if this is what you do to your partner.'

The vaginal examination can be crucial in the diagnosis and treatment of female sexual difficulties. A woman might not consciously admit that she has a problem. The finding of spasm of vaginal muscles by the doctor, when revealed to the woman, allows her to talk about it. The woman is encouraged to examine her vagina with her fingers and to talk about it while she is doing so. The purpose of this is to help her reveal and understand her fantasies about her vagina and her own sexuality. Kaplan (1974) encourages the partner to examine the vagina, and Masters & Johnson (1966) advocate the use of dilators. However, neither of these approaches helps the woman deal with her own fantasies about the vagina. It is understandable that women should have fantasies about their bodies since their sex organs are hidden away. Girls are also often admonished by their mothers if they do try to explore themselves. The doctor's role is thus often that of a good permissive parent allowing the woman to own and be proud of her sexual organs and feelings. Belief that the vagina is 'too small' can also refer to the woman herself: that she is not grown up enough for sex. Women are often disgusted and ashamed of their sexual desires and may refuse to touch the vagina or refer to it as 'a lump of meat' or 'a hole'. Women often believe that they urinate through the vagina. Some think they have a hidden penis in the vagina. Treatment cannot progress unless these fantasies are explored. This method of treatment has been particularly successful with problems of non-consummation, spasm of vaginal muscles and painful intercourse.

The 'Balint' approach together with an account of successfully treated cases has been given by various authors (see Courtenay 1968, Friedman 1962, Tunnadine 1970, Mears 1978). There are about 200 doctors (mainly female) trained and they now belong, since family planning clinics were taken over by the NHS, to the Institute of Psychosexual Medicine. There are about sixty psychosexual clinics; the majority are now run by the NHS and are free. About four patients or couples are seen in a session. About 400 doctors are in training.

Masters & Johnson techniques

The treatment using Masters & Johnson techniques is called 'sex therapy'. It has three basic aims:
  (1)   to clear up myths and misinformation;
  (2)   to lessen anxiety (as previously mentioned, a concomitant of all sexual problems);
  (3)   to facilitate and enhance communication between partners, particularly about sex.
Co-therapists are used, male and female — considered essential by Masters and Johnson in order to have an advocate for each sex. Later workers (e.g. Kaplan 1974) have modified these techniques and use only one therapist. The couple are seen both together (conjoint therapy) and individually.

Outline of treatment

An extensive sexual history of both partners is taken in order to ascertain attitudes, feelings, values with regard to sex and previous sexual experience. Information is then given to clear up myths and misinformation.

The couple are advised *not* to have intercourse but to concentrate on 'pleasuring' (stroking and caressing each other without touching the genitals or breasts). This is 'sensate focusing'. It is considered essential to lessen sexual anxiety. It takes the emphasis off achievement and lessens the anxiety of 'spectatoring', i.e. the person looking down on himself to see how he is performing. It also helps the couple become aware of their own bodies and of their partners', and aids communication, since the couple are requested to tell each other what they like. So often in our culture sex is seen as a wholly genital activity rather than a sensual or sensuous one. Thus sensate focusing helps the person to become aware of his bodily feelings. Sensate focusing can also perform a diagnostic task. One partner may not want the therapy to succeed and may sabotage therapy by refusing to tell the other what he/she likes. Once the sensate focusing is successful, specific techniques are taught for different types of problem. These have been modified by other workers, notably Kaplan. Masters and Johnson originally advised a three-week residential course of treatment. This is now eleven days.

Specific Masters & Johnson treatments for sexual disorders

Impotence   Intercourse and ejaculation are forbidden. The couple concentrate on taking turns in caressing each other and in teasing caresses of the genitals. Later the woman is instructed to caress the penis until it becomes erect; she then stops until the erection is lost and then resumes caressing again. When intercourse is resumed it is initially with the woman in the superior position. Hormones such as testosterone have a limited use and may be used to break the vicious circle of failure by restoring confidence in the ability to have erections. Masters and Johnson claimed a 74% success rate in cases of secondary impotence out of a total of 213 cases. The prognosis is not so good for primary impotence, as this is more likely to be associated with more serious psychiatric disturbances. Cooper (1971) in a review of the treatment of impotence found that brief treatment that focussed on the symptom was more successful than lengthy insight therapy.

Premature ejaculation   A similar approach is used with the woman again caressing the penis with the man lying on his back. He concentrates on the sensation produced and tells her when ejaculation is imminent; she then stops. Caressing is then repeated. Intercourse is eventually resumed with the woman in the superior position astride the man. This is the Semans method advocated in 1956 by J. Semans, a urologist. The approach advocated by Masters and Johnson is the *squeeze technique*. The woman again caresses the penis but this time when the man feels that the climax is imminent the woman squeezes the penis at the junction of the glans with the shaft of the penis so that the man loses his erection. Masters and Johnson reported a 98 per cent success rate with 186 men using this method.

Ejaculatory incompetence or retarded ejaculation   The couple can engage in mutual or oral stimulation, non-genital pleasuring and teasing genital play. Once a highly aroused state has been reached the penis is inserted into the vagina with strong pelvic thrusts. Masters and Johnson reported that none of seventeen patients so treated relapsed after five years.

Female: lack of sexual interest   Sensate focusing is used first, followed by teasing genital play. When the woman has reached a high state of arousal, intercourse takes place. The woman initiates intercourse and also controls the thrusting against the erect penis. She is in the superior position. If the man feels near to orgasm the couple are advised to stop and then re-start. This approach improves many women's sexual responsiveness. However, women with severe conflicts or deep hostility are not helped.

Female: lack of orgasm   The woman is advised to masturbate. This can produce considerable anxiety and attitudes to masturbation have to be dealt with in the therapeutic sessions. A vibrator can be used if a woman needs intense stimulation, though its persistent use is not advocated because there is a danger that she may be unable to achieve orgasm without it. Sometimes women may believe that orgasm may change them and make them promiscuous; others fear the loss of control. Thus some women may fear success. The woman has to be re-assured that orgasm will not change her life dramatically. When the time to achieve orgasm is shorter, the husband can be involved to help his wife have an orgasm, using either a vibrator or his hand. Those women who are conditioned into believing that orgasm must be obtained in intercourse without stimulation of the clitoris may resist such stimulation. This places an enormous burden on the man to keep intercourse going until she can reach orgasm. These women need to work through their guilty feelings about clitoral sensations.

For the treatment of all these conditions it will be noted that cooperation of both partners is essential. This presumes that there are no deep-seated conflicts, resentments or hostilities between the couple. If the partner refuses to cooperate or sabotages treatment, failure will result if this is not dealt with. It may be necessary on these occasions to stop the sex therapy and treat the individual or the relationship.

The remarkable success rates Masters and Johnson achieved with all types of sexual dysfunctions and maintained over five years have not been produced by others (Wright *et al.* 1977). Indeed, the only comparable British study (Bancroft 1976) using modified Masters & Johnson techniques showed only a 37 per cent successful outcome in 97 patients who completed treatment, though another 31 per cent (of the 97) had had a worthwhile improvement. The main reasons for this are that the 510 couples seen by Masters and Johnson were highly selected, well motivated, with a good marital relationship. Couples had to reside in a hotel in St Louis during treatment and everything was done to make their stay a happy one (analogous to a second honeymoon) so that they were protected from the daily wear and tear of family life. Those couples who sought treatment and who lived in St Louis did less well than those who came from outside St Louis. Masters and Johnson discuss their treatment failures. These mainly occurred where the marriages were on the point of breaking up and one of the partners or both sabotaged treatment, others were 'therapeutic nihilists', — people who had had all kinds of treatment including prolonged psychotherapy.

Although Masters & Johnson techniques have been described as behaviourist, they themselves deny this and state that the techniques are of little or no value without supportive psychotherapy for the marital relationship.

The relationship and the interaction of the couple are the primary focus of treatment. Where couples were already undergoing psychotherapy, Masters and Johnson only concentrated on the sexual difficulty with emphasis on re-education.

The present position in Britain regarding Masters & Johnson techniques

Masters & Johnson techniques are beginning to be used more widely by psychosexual doctors belonging to the Institute of Psychosexual Medicine, several psychiatric departments in NHS hospitals, some marriage guidance counsellors, and private therapists. Perhaps a note of caution should be struck here. In the United States Masters and Johnson at a recent conference expressed anxieties about the professional competence of some 'sex therapists' using their techniques. While it is true that many sexual difficulties are of a superficial nature needing only

re-education, others are more complex with psychological conflicts in one or both partners together with relationship and
marital difficulties, and these may need to be treated either
before or in conjunction with the sexual problem.

Other approaches

Films, books and sexual aids such as vibrators have been used
by some workers in conjunction with Masters and Johnson
techniques in order to free couples from their inhibitions and to
give them permission to explore their own sexual fantasies and
what excites them (Gillan 1977).

Couples groups Couples with sexual difficulties are brought
together to talk and share their problems.

Surrogate partners The use of surrogate partners, male or
female, is a contentious one and they are used at only one
centre, the Institute of Sex Education & Research in
Birmingham. Masters and Johnson used female surrogates for
sexually dysfunctional unmarried men (men who had impotence or premature ejaculation). They found that the surrogate partner was extremely useful for the man but not the
woman, since they believed that women considered warmth
and emotional response more important than effective sexual
functioning. The reason postulated for this is that a man, to be
effective for procreation, has to be potent, in contrast to the
woman where effective sexual functioning is not required for
her to become a mother. One of the dangers in the use of surrogates is the emotional involvement of one of the partners. It
would also be possible for the man to be potent with a surrogate but not with other women.

Feminist therapy groups These help women to become comfortable with their own bodies. Help is given with self-examination. Masturbatory techniques are taught in the pre-orgasmic
groups which have had some success in the United States.

Behaviourist techniques Systematic desensitisation techniques have been used to treat impotence, premature ejaculation and lack of interest in sex in the woman. Patients are
trained in relaxation techniques to help overcome anxiety. They
are then encouraged to lie beside their partners and begin love
play. If this is successful, they are encouraged to increase the
amount of sex play but on no account to attempt intercourse
until all anxiety has been relieved. This is called a 'system of
hierarchies', a step-by-step procedure until intercourse is

established. Many behaviourists insist on tailor-made programmes to suit the individual rather than applying the same techniques to everyone. For example, the husband who avoids confrontation and argument and who may well be impotent can be helped to assert himself. This is done by means of role play with the therapist. The man then practises at home with his wife. One drawback is that the wife is expected to cooperate, and where she does not want to relinquish her role as the dominant partner the treatment of itself will hardly be successful!

Marital contract therapy This refers to helping the couple who are always criticising each other and finding fault to say positive things to each other. Each partner is asked to list what they want the other to do or be like. Their requests have to be specific, thus 'I would like my husband to kiss me every night when he comes home from work' rather than 'I want him to love me'. An agreement is then reached that where one partner does something the other wants he or she in turn receives a specified reward. Although these techniques have been criticised as being too superficial, proponents say that couples learn about their own destructive behaviour and how this affects the relationship.

SOME ILLUSTRATIVE CASES OF TREATMENT OF SEXUAL DYSFUNCTION

1 *Guilt about premarital sex*

Mr and Mrs A. attended a psychosexual doctor referred by their GP. The complaint was painful intercourse. Mrs A. also complained of headaches and stomach-aches and was awaiting hospital investigation for these. Mrs A. was well dressed in a rather severe way with gloves, hat and umbrella. Mr A., more casually dressed, was angry and resentful. It later emerged that he had developed premature ejaculation in order to get intercourse over quickly after Mrs A's complaints of pain. Exploration of the guilt surrounding their premarital activities (they were both strict Catholics and had a 'lovely white wedding') together with vaginal examination and self-examination with permission by a parent figure to be sexual resulted in a cure after three sessions. The hospital appointment was cancelled. Mr A's premature ejaculation also ceased.

2 *Unrealised marital expectations*

Mr and Mrs B. attended a clinic: the complaint was lack of interest in sex, possibly due to the pill, that was leading to quarrels. Both had married with a romantic view of life. She would be the good little wife — washing, ironing, cooking, etc., like her mother. He would be the good husband and never quarrel as he had seen his parents do. The romance turned sour when she found that he so enjoyed being waited on 'hand and foot' that he was not prepared to help her when she was tired. (She also had a full-time job.) Whenever she tried to tell him about it he would hide behind a book. They could not have a good row. Her resentment spilled over to the sexual side, hence her lack of interest. Exploration of the marital relationship together with Masters & Johnson techniques led to a successful result in six sessions.

3 *Denial of sexuality as a result of parental sexual problems*

Miss C. attended a clinic where spasm of the vaginal muscles was discovered on routine examination. She refused to examine herself. She was seen regularly over the course of a year. Her parents had fought when she was a child over money and sex. (Her mother wanted the money: her father the sex.) Mother kept Miss C in bed with her and she witnessed repeated scenes of father coming to mother wanting sex, which mother refused 'because of her daughter'. Miss C believed that she had denied mother a sexual life and must punish herself by denying herself one. Father's visits had also made her excited but afraid, so while she could allow herself to get excited (she had had many boyfriends) she could not 'let them in' vaginally. When told that if mother and father had really wanted sex she could not have stopped them it enabled her to give herself permission to have sex herself.

4 *The girl-wife and the fear of sex*

This case illustrates how the solution to one problem can unmask another where the balance of a collusive relationship has been upset.

Mrs D. was overweight but pretty, in her early twenties, and cried a great deal during the first interview. She presented with a lack of interest in sex. She had married a much older man and though she liked to think of herself as very mature, behaved in many ways like a little girl looking for love. It emerged that her parents had been divorced and that she had been brought up by a grandmother who had died recently. The loss of interest in sex dated from that time. Mrs D.'s husband was invited to attend for one interview. He was a big, quiet man who seemed uninvolved in the proceedings apart from patting his wife's hand every few minutes as if she were a small child. The doctor focused on Mrs D.'s relationship with her grandmother, feeling that her death had not been properly mourned. Many tearful sessions then ensued and although Mrs D. really seemed to have worked through the mourning, sex did not improve. The doctor, feeling at a loss, decided that Mrs D.'s family tree might provide some clues about views on sex. It emerged from the family tree that women (apart from her strict grandmother) tended to be 'flighty', leaving husbands, taking lovers, as indeed her own mother had done. Once it was explained to Mrs D. that to be sexy did not mean that she would become flighty and unfaithful, sex improved rapidly. Mrs D. seemed to grow up overnight. This had profound consequences, particularly when she talked of having children (previously they had decided against having children). The husband then began to be unable to ejaculate intravaginally. His need for a girl-wife and his fear of parenthood were unmasked by his wife's cure.

5 Premature ejaculation and an unfaithful husband

Mr E, a 35-year-old married man with two children presented with premature ejaculation and secondary impotence. His penis was 'weak' and the fluid 'ran away'. He seemed anxious to please and rather ingratiating, but also sad. When this was commented on he related how he had had an affair two years before while his wife was in hospital with a difficult pregnancy. His wife subsequently discovered this. She at first refused to have sex with him. Later, after repeated assurances from the husband that the affair was at an end, she relented. However, now she watched him minutely during every sex act and if he did not get erect quickly she accused him of having another affair. Her anger and resentment at what he had done vented themselves in disparaging remarks about his penis. She frequently commented that she could no longer 'feel him inside'. The wife attended the second interview. She was pretty but overweight and regarded the doctor (female) suspiciously. Comment about this led to an angry outpouring about her husband's affair. The doctor recognises the pain and hurt behind the anger and commented upon it. The wife then started to talk about her weight and how unattractive she felt. She believed her husband was always making comparisons between her and his former girlfriend. Discussion about this, during which the husband reiterated his love, together with explanations about how his anxiety about her watching and testing him resulted in his premature ejaculation seemed to lead to a relaxation in her attitudes. Subsequent sessions using Masters & Johnson techniques (sensate focusing and squeeze technique) led to a complete cure with both partners stressing how they could really 'feel' the penis once again.

THE SOCIAL WORKER AND SEXUAL PROBLEMS

Few social workers are at present trained to be sex therapists or psychosexual counsellors. For the majority of social workers, therefore, the important issues will centre around finding out whether there is a sexual problem and deciding what to do about it once it is discovered. This may be complicated either because there are no local agencies to help (or the client refuses to attend) or because there is such a plethora that it is difficult for the social worker to know which agency is best for his client's particular problem.

Discovering the problem

This will depend on the social worker and the client and their relationship.

The social worker Social workers will have varying degrees of comfort in discussing sex with their clients. The clients themselves will be sensitive to any discomfort on the part of the social worker and this may inhibit them from revealing the true nature of their difficulties. Thus the social worker should first of all try to make himself comfortable talking about sex. This, of course, is made easier by experience. It may sound facile, but one possible approach is for the social worker to practise a few stock questions about sex (preferably in front of a mirror until he is quite relaxed), such as 'Is everything all right with the physical/sexual side of your relationship/marriage?' 'Do you have any problems with sex relations?' The client is thereby given permission to talk about sex. The questions should be introduced casually as merely one aspect of enquiry into the client's life. This is less threatening than introducing it as a problem area. A note of caution needs to be sounded. The fact that nowadays people do feel more able to talk about and admit to a sexual problem may deter the social worker from looking at other problems that the client may have, yet feel are too painful to reveal. For example, a woman with depression complained she had no interest in sex. The depression could have been blamed for this but in fact she was found to be punishing herself for an abortion she had had two years previously which she had not fully mourned. Once help was given with this the sex problem resolved itself. Part of the comfort in talking about sex will be for the social worker to familiarise himself with the words that clients use for sex and related matters. This is not to say that the social worker needs to resort to four-letter words all the time, but he must convey that he does understand what the client means. By telling the client the medical terms he can provide him with a vocabulary that can be used publicly; for example, when seeing the doctor or attending a clinic.

The client   As discussed earlier, the sexual problem can be masked as a contraceptive, medical, marital, child or family problem, and only by gentle and sensitive questioning can the real problem be discovered. In all cases where there are problems with children, whether babies, toddlers or adolescents, the social worker should be alert to marital and sexual difficulties. Housing problems, particularly sharing with in-laws and lack of privacy, may initiate or exacerbate sexual difficulties.

Worries and stress of any kind are likely to depress sexual functions.

Fertility may affect sexual function, that is where a pregnancy is desperately wanted or where there is an unintended and unwanted pregnancy. This issue will be dealt with in more detail in Part 2. Venereal disease with resultant broken trust can also lead to sexual difficulties. This too is examined in subsequent chapters.

The seduction issue

There is an understandable anxiety about seduction, whenever sexual problems are raised — whether the social worker will be accused by the client's spouse of attempting to seduce the client, especially where they are of opposite sex; or the client himself may so accuse the social worker. The social worker may be concerned about the involvement of his own feelings, being sexually attracted to the client and vice versa. There is the difficulty of the sexually provocative teenager, particularly of the nubile teenage girl and the young male social worker. This issue is ever-present in residential homes together with a constant worry of false accusations reaching the newspaper headlines. (The teenager and sex will be considered later.) Where there is anxiety concerning false accusations by possibly hysterical and manipulative clients it may be wiser for the social worker to interview them in the office rather than at home.

Feelings of sexual attraction will be inevitable from time to time between the social worker and the client (as of course between doctor and patient). The social worker ought to be able to acknowledge this attraction. Indeed, this often has a beneficial effect for the person who feels sexually unattractive, but the social worker needs to make it perfectly clear by his manner or words where the boundaries lie and that they will not be crossed. There is, after all, an enormous difference between having feelings and putting them into action. The personal integrity of both social worker and client needs to be sacrosanct. It is unfortunately true that in the United States in the name of therapy, some professional helpers have taken advantage of their position to have sex with their clients, a practice firmly denounced by Masters and Johnson.

What to do with the sexual problem where referral is not possible

It must be remembered that in over 50 per cent of cases of sexual dysfunction both partners are affected, so this should determine whether both partners are seen or referred for help. Where the client refuses to attend a clinic (and this does happen where the client is too shy or embarrassed to repeat his story all over again) or where there is no local specialised help available, there is still much that the social worker can do.

(1) He can correct any misunderstandings or misinformation, remembering that sexual difficulties can be due to ignorance. This is particularly pertinent to working-class clients and to clients from different ethnic backgrounds.

(2) He can be the 'good' parent encouraging the client to express his sexual feelings and admit his sexual interests and

desires and thus allow him to be sexual, remembering that the cause of the client's difficulty may be in the failure of the latter's parents to give him permission. This cannot be emphasised enough, since the parent's role, especially that of the opposite-sex parent, in affirming the sexuality of the child is perhaps the single most important factor determining a person's attitude to his own sexuality.

(3) Sexual difficulties are compounded and caused by poor communication. The social worker can act as an intermediary, helping the couple discuss and share their difficulties.

(4) The use of Masters & Johnson techniques by the social worker untrained in sexual counselling is perhaps controversial. The social worker runs the risk of getting out of his depth and disillusioning the couple about the efficacy of sex therapy. The biggest pitfall is the quality of the couple's relationship. For Masters & Johnson techniques to work this has to be good, without any underlying hostility and resentment that could sabotage treatment. One way of testing whether this exists is to suggest the sensate focusing technique; that is, for the couple to spend time each evening, say 20–30 minutes for about one to two weeks, caressing and stroking each other in turn in a non-demanding way i.e. without the expectation of sexual intercourse. Failure to do this usually exposes the under-lying hostility. Couples may present plausible excuses — not enough time, too many other things to do, too tired. Their motivation may then have to be challenged. Should one partner secretly want to end the marriage or be having an affair, the sensate focusing will be sabotaged. Thus before the social worker attempts to use Masters & Johnson techniques he must ascertain that the relationship is basically a good one.

(5) Since secondary sexual problems are often the result of altered life situations or added stress — loss of work, job pro-motion, money worries, problems with children, ill health — help with these difficulties and explanations of how stress can cause sexual problems may alleviate some of them. A thorough medical check-up may be necessary and the man or woman should be referred to the GP.

Referral

Referring properly is a skill which is often not taught in medical and social work courses. The success of treatment may depend on how a referral is made and whether referral is appropriate.

Referral is too often made as an easy way out of a painful (to the worker) situation. There is a tendency to use an agency as a 'dumping ground' for difficult or unpleasant cases on the basis of 'leaving no stone unturned'. Referral can be seen by the client as rejection unless the reasons for it are carefully gone into. Some workers find it difficult to refer since the need to do so makes them feel inept. Thus there are problems with 'letting go' and accepting that what can be done has been done. Sharing care is another fraught area — this is looked at in Part 2.

Some guidelines on referral for sexual difficulties

a) Get to know the agency/personnel who are offering treatment.
b) Find out what kind of treatment is given, e.g. Masters & Johnson, behavioural approaches, psychosexual counselling or an eclectic approach.
c) Find out whether therapy is given by a single therapist or co-therapists.
d) Find out whether the individual is treated, or the couple are always seen together, or whether a more flexible approach is used.
e) Find out the possible length of treatment, the kind of commitment required of the client and whether this can be realistically fitted in with work requirements, care of children, etc.
g) Find out how to refer — direct referral by the social worker, self-referral or referral through the GP.

The client needs to be prepared for the experience and what will be required of him. It may be appropriate for the social worker to continue seeing the client while he attends the therapist. This will need to be clarified with the therapist to avoid competition or manipulation by the client.

A directory of agencies offering help with psychosexual problems has been produced by the British Association for Counselling (BAC). It covers most of Britain. However, it is not exhaustive. Information is provided on means of referral, kinds of therapy offered, training background and whether a fee is necessary. Information about local psychosexual clinics run by doctors trained by the Institute of Psychosexual Medicine is usually available from family planning clinics. Hospital departments providing help with sexual problems usually require referral by the GP. Referral to the Marriage Guidance Council can be direct by the social worker or by self-referral. Treatment from psychosexual clinics run by the National Health Service and from the Marriage Guidance Council is free.

3
Sex and the Handicapped

Attitudes towards the sexuality of the physically and mentally handicapped have until recently been extremely negative. Since both groups to a lesser or greater extent need care from the community there is a tendency to regard the handicapped rather in the light of children. Thus as children are not supposed to have a sex life, then neither should the handicapped. They are not and cannot be sexual people. Associated with these somewhat irrational attitudes are very real anxieties about the capabilities of the handicapped in caring for a husband or wife and for children. The parents of handicapped young people often experience great difficulty in accepting that they have sexual feelings and needs. Anxiety about sexual exploitation which may well have a realistic basis leads them to be too protective. The handicapped have tended to accept this. However, there are signs, due to the work of the SPOD Committee (Sexual Problems of the Disabled), the Family Planning Association and individual doctors, psychologists and social workers, that the situation is changing. Furthermore, the handicapped themselves are beginning to express their feelings about this area of their lives (see BBC TV film 'Like other people' which depicts a spastic couple). Sex education for the handicapped is extremely variable in quantity and quality and may be absent altogether. As with other areas of sexuality, the social worker will have to examine his own attitudes with regard to sex and the handicapped. Professional careers have tended to reflect society's negative attitudes. There has also been a lack of training in this area.

THE PHYSICALLY HANDICAPPED

There are possibly over 400,000 physically handicapped people between the ages of 16 and 65. This number includes those whose limbs are disabled, those who are blind or deaf and those who have multiple handicaps. The blind number about 97,000 and the deaf form 3—4 per cent of the population. Thus the range of problems is vast and complex. The person handicapped from birth faces a different situation to that of the person who becomes handicapped in middle life. The medical profession, to its shame, has largely ignored the sexual needs of the handicapped and, indeed, may know little about them and how best to help.

A committee on sexual problems of the disabled (SPOD) was set up in 1973 by the National Fund for Research into Crippling Diseases, to study and advise on sexual problems as these might occur among disabled people. A study of the sexual problems of physically disabled people carried out on behalf of the committee in 1974-5 by the Research Institute for Communal Affairs showed clearly that the majority of disabled people encounter sexual problems associated with their disability and, disturbingly, that any thorough knowledge of the problems and of solutions to them is rare in the helping professions.

The survey carried out was on 212 disabled people living in Coventry and revealed that half had *current* sexual problems. The incidence was greater in men than in women.

There were four main areas of difficulties:
a) potency problems;
b) difficulties with physical comfort;
c) difficulties with sexual movements and postures;
d) emotional relationship problems.
Disabled people were less frequently married than the general population and marriage breakdown was more common.

The physically handicapped can be divided into two main groups (Hamilton 1978):

a) those in whom sexual function is potentially normal but the expression of it may be made difficult by physical discomfort, pain, muscle spasm and/or weakness, limb deformity, and involuntary movement;

b) those with abnormal sexual function caused by the illness itself or drugs given to treat the illness.

The first group includes those with chronic illness such as arthritis, heart and lung disease, cerebral palsy, muscular dystrophy and multiple sclerosis in its early stages. The blind, deaf and dumb are also included.

The second group includes those with spinal cord damage, spina bifida, multiple sclerosis in its later stages and diabetes. In these conditions the ability of the male to have or maintain an erection may be lost and the normal sequence of ejaculation and accompanying orgasm may not take place. Sterility is common in the male. The female may be able to have intercourse and become pregnant but may be unable to experience orgasm.

As well as the physical symptoms of pain, fatigue, muscle spasm and so on there are also psychological difficulties. The disabled person may feel sexually unattractive and even disgusting, there may be a fear of being rebuffed, or damaged or of passing on an inherited disease. Shame and guilt may be experienced for having sexual desires and needs, especially if these cannot be satisfied in the 'normal' way in the 'normal' position, i.e. sexual intercourse with the man on top. The disabled often find it difficult to meet partners and to ensure privacy if and when they do. As they often have to be physically carried, washed and changed they cannot own their genitals in the same way as those who are not handicapped. Looking after the handicapped may be embarrassing and so there is a tendency to keep physical contact to the minimum and to carry it out with mechanical efficiency.

The blind have particular problems. The sighted rely on vision for sexual stimulation. The blind have to rely on sound, smell and touch which involve more intimate contact. As children they cannot experiment in the sex play of sighted children because they can never be sure that they are not being spied upon. The body changes of puberty can be alarming, especially as there can be no reassuring mirror. Blind girls tend to menstruate earlier and have to rely on smell and symptoms to inform them when their periods have begun. The blind girl always has the worry that her periods will begin without her knowing it. Sex education for the blind poses special problems. The blind cannot conceive of the shape and size of the genital organs or breasts without feeling them. They should be encouraged to explore their own bodies. In Sweden live models are used. The repertoire of subtle exchanges, for example, in glances or voice tone so important for sexual courtship is denied to those with visual and hearing defects.

What can be done to help

For some disabled people the handicaps may be so great that very little practical help can be given. However, fantasy plays a large part in the sex lives of most people and the handicapped are no exception. They should be encouraged in this. Sharing one's difficulties and disappointments with an attentive and concerned person can also be beneficial in itself. The social worker will need to be prepared to initiate discussions on sex with the disabled client. It may be necessary, also, to help the parents of a disabled child, particularly the adolescent, to recognise and accept that their child is also a sexual person and to encourage them to teach their children how to masturbate. Alternative ways of making love such as body caressing, mutual masturbation or oral sex should be discussed where intercourse is not possible. So often where intercourse is regarded as the only way to express sexuality these other ways are regarded as 'perversions' or 'not quite nice' or 'not right'. Discussion by a professional worker can sanction such activity. Special care may need to be paid to personal hygiene to prevent the risk of infection, especially where the handicapped person has bladder and bowel problems, so advice from a specialist may be necessary.

Use of different positions   Intercourse may be difficult with the man on top. Alternative positions can be suggested such as the woman astride the man, or the man entering the woman from behind or the couple lying on their side either face to face or with the man behind the woman. Cushions and pillows placed under the back can raise the hips so that penetration can be made easier. They can also be used to support painful or weak limbs or lessen muscle spasm.

Sexual aids   There are many sexual aids now available. A free catalogue can be obtained from Blakoe Ltd (for address, see p. 323). Sex appliances can be prescribed on the NHS, but only by hospital consultants.

Vibrators   These are battery operated and can be used by both men and women to obtain orgasms. They are particularly useful for those who get tired or breathless easily or who have limited use of their hands.

Penile prostheses   Some can be fitted on to a semi-erect penis, others can be strapped on and are fitted with vibrators. If sexual aids are to be used, the couple should be counselled together to ensure that both partners find their use acceptable.

Contraceptive advice   may be needed. The couple can be referred (or taken) to a family planning clinic or general practitioner (see Part 2).

Genetic counselling   may be required where there is the possibility of passing on the handicap. Referral to a specialist centre will need to be done by the general practitioner.

Psychological problems The difficulties encountered may vary according to whether one or both partners are disabled, whether the disability came before or after marriage and whether the marriage was a stable one before the disability. Unfortunately, when the disability occurs in one partner after marriage there is a much higher chance of break-up. Chronic illness or disability may be used as an excuse not to have sex, especially where sex is regarded as sinful or distasteful. There may also be a fear that sex will make the disability worse. If the partner is able-bodied there may be fears of damaging the handicapped partner, or the handicapped partner may be no longer regarded as sexually attractive or exciting. This can happen where the disability occurs after marriage. Disability occurring in this way often leads to anger and depression, which in turn can lead to sexual difficulties such as impotence or lack of response in the woman.

Agencies providing help There are few special clinics providing help solely for disabled people with sexual difficulties. However, SPOD does provide an advisory and counselling service for disabled people experiencing sexual difficulties. It also provides an information service for professional and voluntary workers with the disabled regarding local facilities for counselling. Certain disabilities have their own special society such as the Spastics Society for those with cerebral palsy and the Multiple Sclerosis Society for sufferers from that disease, which give guidance with sexual difficulties. Psychosexual counselling clinics and family planning clinics, both run by the Area Health Authorities for the NHS, and the Marriage Guidance Council also provide information, advice and counselling for the disabled.

The staff in some residential homes for the severely handicapped are beginning to help the disabled with masturbation and with intercourse if the couple need it. The decision to do this has many inherent difficulties — the effect on the staff and their own relationships and the danger of exploitation of the disabled who may be unable to protect themselves. It should only be resorted to if the individual members of the staff wish to be so involved and if there are staff discussions and support available for them. Given the present position of the law and the disabled, it would seem advisable that if sexual 'assistance' is given to a person in a residential home, it should be provided by a female member of staff on whom no prohibition exists under the Sexual Offences Acts 1956 and 1967. Consent of the disabled is essential. Further advice concerning the legal aspects of sex and the disabled is available from SPOD.

THE MENTALLY HANDICAPPED

There are about 110,000 severely subnormal people (IQ below 50) of whom about 60,000 are in residential care. There are about 350,000 mildly sub-normal people (IQ 50–70). Four children in every thousand suffer from severe mental handicap: rates are higher for the milder form. The majority of mentally handicapped children have parents who are within the average range of intelligence. The main causes of mental handicap are brain damage and mongolism (Down's Syndrome).

The mentally handicapped unaffected by physical handicaps do not usually have any problems with sexual functioning, apart from those caused by ignorance and fear. It is unfortunate that certain myths relating to sexuality and the handicapped have been used to prevent the giving of information about sex. These myths are as follows:
   a) the mentally handicapped have no sexual desires;
   b) they are 'sex maniacs' and have insatiable desires;
   c) they are sexually deviant;
   d) they are incapable of dealing with sex responsibly.
Denied information, the change of adolescence may come as a shock. The adolescent boy experiencing frequent erections will begin to masturbate and will do this in public if he is not given guidance. Recent discussions with the staff of an adult training centre for the mentally handicapped revealed that masturbation in public was a common problem. Many of the staff found it embarrassing and would either ignore it or attempt to distract the person. Only a few felt comfortable enough to discuss masturbation openly with the person concerned and offer appropriate guidance, i.e. that there is nothing wrong or dirty about masturbation but that it should be done in private. Masturbation may be the only way in which the handicapped person, particularly the severely handicapped, can express his sexuality. Ignoring the sexuality of the handicapped may lead to sexual behaviour such as exposing the genitals or masturbating in public places, which may bring the person into unnecessary and painful contact with the law. This only reinforces the view that the handicapped are sexually deviant. The protective attitudes of both parents and professional carers are under-

standable — handicapped persons (depending on the degree of handicap) may have poor judgement and never reach emotional maturity. They may do whatever is asked of them without questioning. They also tend to give affection indiscriminately. Girls, in particular, may respond to sexual attention and are at risk from sexual exploitation. It is this which possibly gives handicapped girls the reputation of being promiscuous. Some handicapped girls, particularly if they are not in a supportive and caring environment, may be tempted into prostitution. For all these reasons the giving of information about sex and preparation for dealing with sexual relationships, including contraception, is of vital importance. Ideally this sex education should involve the parents, the professional careers and the handicapped themselves. The social worker with his intimate knowledge of the handicapped person and his family is often in a key position to facilitate a change in attitudes and to provide simple, straightforward information. He can also be the link between the care staff in residential homes and training centres and the parents.

Some handicapped people may wish to marry and have children. This may occasion great anxiety, particularly for the parents. It used to be feared (and this led to the segregation of the sexes among the mentally handicapped) that the handicapped would by reason of their alleged greater fertility eventually outbreed the more intelligent. While a minority of the mentally handicapped may have very large families, the majority may either have 1 to 2 children or none at all. The IQ of the offspring if both parents are mentally retarded is likely to be low but not as low as the parents' (De la Cruz & La Veck 1973, Hilliard 1968). How well the handicapped married couple will cope with children will depend on their living standards and the support they are given, particularly with regard to family planning. Thus adequate spacing between children (say 3—4 years) and limiting their number to two or three may enable the handicapped couple to cope with the minimum of outside help (see Chapter 13). That many such mildly sub-normal couples can cope adequately given proper support and guidance has been demonstrated already (Craft M. & A. 1978). Indeed, the couple may manage far better with housekeeping etc. together than they could as individuals living separately since one partner may compensate for the deficiencies in the other (De la Cruz & La Veck 1973). Organisations already in existence which can help the handicapped in relationship to sexual

and contraceptive matters are the Marriage Guidance Council
and family planning clinics.

4

Homosexuality

HOMOSEXUALITY AND THE SOCIAL WORKER

Social workers will need to be aware of their own attitudes and feelings regarding homosexuality since these will determine the care they give to homosexuals. For some social workers (as with other professionals) homosexuality may pose a threat to their own sexual self-image, or they may have incorporated society's attitudes towards homosexuals and have preconceived ideas about them. The dangers of this discomfort will be:

a) to reinforce the negative self-image that homosexuals tend to have;

b) to attempt to change the homosexual without regard to his feelings and wishes.

The social worker may himself be homosexual. This can pose other problems. He may be fearful of discovery or he may see the solutions to his own difficulties as applicable to those of the person seeking help. The homosexual social worker may experience difficulty in understanding heterosexual problems, particularly in relation to family planning and the stresses that contraception can place upon a sexual relationship.

DEFINITION AND INCIDENCE

Confusion appears to exist in defining homosexuality. For some it refers only to physical sexual acts (usually anal intercourse); to others it is an emotional and psychological preference for the same sex which may or may not be accompanied by sexual acts. Kinsey's findings (Kinsey *et al*. 1948) challenged the view that there were two kinds of sexual people, namely heterosexual and homosexual. Evidence was found for a continuum of hetero-sexuality—homosexuality. Kinsey found that 60 per cent of all boys (Kinsey *et al*. 1948) and 33 per cent of girls (Kinsey *et al*. 1953) have engaged in at least one act of overtly homosexual sex play by the age of fifteen. 37 per cent of the male and 13 per cent of the female population engage at one time in their lives in some form of homosexual activity leading to orgasm; 8 per cent of men have been exclusively homosexual for a period of at least three years and 4 per cent have been homosexual all their lives; 13 per cent of men admitted to homosexual feelings but no overt experience. Only half of Kinsey's male sample were exclusively heterosexual; 72 per cent of the female sample were so. Kinsey's figures were based on acts, or outlets, as he termed them, and did not involve emotional or psychological involvement. Kinsey believed his figures to be accurate regarding the *kind* of behaviour reported but not the frequency — that is, people are more likely to remember what they have done rather than the number of times they did it. Subsequent studies, though on much smaller samples, have revealed similar findings. (Weinberg & Williams 1974, Spencer 1959, Ross 1950). Although Kinsey's research revealed that certain individuals engage in both heterosexual and homosexual activities (wrongly termed bisexuality, which, in biological terms, refers to animals having both the anatomy and the functions of both sexes, e.g. the earthworm). Some writers (Hertoft 1976, Babuscio 1977) believe that in practice it is possible to classify a person as hetero or homosexual. The latest study from the Institute for Sex Research (founded by Kinsey) shows that a fairly strong heterosexual element was found in about a third of the homosexual men studied (Bell & Weinberg 1978). This heterosexual element could take the form of heterosexual dreams, fantasies, or actual arousal in a heterosexual situation. Despite this, only 20 per cent of this sample actually married. In the majority of these cases the marriage broke up, mainly as a result of homosexual involvement. It would seem important in view of these findings that individuals should not feel pressurised by society to marry in order to 'prove' either to themselves or to others that they are 'normal'. One may hope that when the social stigma surrounding homosexuality is removed, people will be enabled to show their true sexual preferences.

THE LAW

The 1967 reform of the 1956 Sexual Offences Act legalised sexual activity in privacy between two consenting males over twenty-one (except in Scotland, Northern Ireland and the Armed Services). There is no legislation regarding the female. A possibly apocryphal story is told to the effect that this is because Queen Victoria could not believe that women engaged in such practices. Despite the change in the law, the homosexual often faces harassment in finding a sexual partner. Examples of this are the police campaigns against clubs or other resorts when they become well known as homosexual meeting places. The homosexual who makes it known that he is one risks dismissal from employment, especially when this involves contact with the young or where he is in a public position.

WHY IS SOCIETY SO ANXIOUS ABOUT HOMOSEXUALITY?

Reference has already been made to Judaeo-Christian concepts and their concern with reproductive sex and hence the unnaturalness of homosexuality which is non-procreative. Once something is labelled unnatural it becomes either a sin to be punished or an illness to be treated. The prevailing twentieth-century view until recently (see American Medical Association 1974 verdict which decided that homosexuality should no longer be considered a psychiatric illness) was that homosexuals were psychologically disturbed or immature and needed treatment. This view is, unfortunately, still held by many analysts and probably by most of the public. The intensity of feeling excited by homosexuality (though the majority of homosexuals are hard working, law-abiding citizens) suggests that what people are really afraid of is the extent to which homosexual feelings exist in themselves. Sadly the married homosexuals, who either deny their homosexual experiences or who are fearful of exposure, are often those who attack homosexuality most vehemently. A further anxiety about homosexuality is the confusion between it and paedophilia. While some homosexuals — or indeed, heterosexuals — may show a preference for children, the majority do not.

Homosexuality has not been condemned in all societies. 'The majority of human societies condone or even encourage homosexuality for at least some of the population' (Ford & Beach 1951). Homosexuality was accepted between certain individuals at certain times of their lives in ancient Greece. Thus an older married man would court a youth with gifts. Although sexual relations took place the youth was not supposed to enjoy them (Dover 1978). The origins of Greek homosexuality are unknown. One view is that it lay in the need to intensify military bonding.

CAUSES OF HOMOSEXUALITY

Despite the existence of homosexuality for thousands of years and in different societies, it has so far not been possible to explain why some people are homosexual. Perhaps its prolonged existence indicates that it really is a variant of normal sexual behaviour and should in no way be regarded as abnormal. There is no firm evidence that homosexuality is genetically or hormonally determined. Hormone levels affecting the foetal brain may be significant, though there is no definite proof. 'No one has ever succeeded in showing that the general run of homosexuals have any systematic physical variation from the norm for heterosexual man and woman' (West 1976).

Psychological causes and family pattern

Freud suggested a theory of constitutional bisexuality, that is an innate predisposition to the same sex and opposite sex partners. The choice between the two was determined by experiential factors in childhood. Later analysts such as Bieber (1962) and Socarides (1968) have emphasised the experiential factors. According to their view there is guilt and anxiety related to heterosexuality which forces the individual to become homosexual. This guilt and anxiety is caused by a seductive, over-protective mother and a father who is weak or hostile or who is absent from home. The boy is supposed to prefer quiet games, does not care for sports, dislikes fighting and is attached to mother. However, analysts are likely to see only those homosexuals distressed, for whatever reason, by their homosexuality. The fact that many heterosexuals share similar family patterns and a close mother-child relationship would seem to argue against these theories.

It is sometimes thought that homosexuals are different psychologically to heterosexuals. In a widely quoted study (Hooker 1957) experts were unable to distinguish between homosexual or heterosexual men on the basis of their responses to various psychological tests. Other studies have failed to show differences between homosexual and heterosexual individuals on the basis of their psychological adjustment (Chang & Bloch 1960, Saghir & Robins 1973). In the latest study on homosexuality (Bell & Weinberg 1978) homosexuals were divided into five types on the basis of the stability of their relationships and the level of self-acceptance. Only two types were found to be less well adjusted psychologically than heterosexual men. These were the 'dysfunctional' and 'asexual' types who were found to have more regrets about their homosexuality and greater difficulty in finding a suitable partner and maintaining affection. Thus, as the authors themselves state, 'homosexual adults who have come to terms with their homosexuality, who do not regret their sexual orientation and who can function effectively sexually and socially are no more distressed psychologically than are heterosexual men and women'.

Much less is known about female homosexuality (lesbianism), perhaps because it has occasioned less anxiety than male homosexuality. It is often stated that lesbian relationships have a greater emotional component and that such relationships are more stable than those of male homosexuals. It could equally be argued that since the social pressures are not as great against female homosexuality, their relationships are not subjected to the same stress and hence are more stable. Again certain family patterns and parent-child relationships are held responsible, viz. an aggressive or brutal father (or a weak one) with a dominant unloving mother who does not act as a good feminine model.

The seduction theory of causality

One of the anxieties about homosexual teachers, youth leaders, etc. is that they will use their position to seduce young people and turn them into homosexuals. It is sometimes believed that homosexuals become so as a result of seduction. This does not explain how the original homosexuals developed. The seduction theory has been the basis for the higher age limit in law (twenty-one years) for homosexual relations than for heterosexual relations (sixteen years). There is a certain irony here since psychoanalytic theory holds that there is a homosexual phase through which adolescents pass on the way to becoming heterosexual. Babuscio, himself homosexual, appears (1977) to support the view that the conditioning of the first sexual experience with a person of the same sex *is* important to the later development of homosexuality. However, boys who indulge in much homosexual experimentation do not necessarily or even usually develop into homosexual adults (West 1976). Hertoft (1976) agrees with this view and maintains that young people frequently encounter homosexual advances and learn how to deal with them. Most homosexuals describe their first overt experiences as the culmination of previous homosexual fantasies rather than an introduction to something new (West 1976). Stable heterosexuals do not change even after quite extensive homosexual experience, e.g. in prison (Gibbons 1957).

Thus the causes of homosexuality (if, indeed, there are any) are not known for certain. What is clear is that, given the intense feelings both for and against homosexuality as a variant of normal sexual behaviour, objectivity is difficult to maintain.

Whatever view is taken of homosexuality and its causes, the misery and suffering of homosexuals past and present, due to societal attitudes, is undoubted and unnecessary. Perhaps the most important issue concerning homosexuality (as with heterosexuality) is the quality of the relationships. The evidence so far available shows that they can be as deep and enduring or as superficial and casual as heterosexual ones.

SEXUAL BEHAVIOUR OF HOMOSEXUALS

Male homosexuals practise mutual masturbation, oral sex (fellatio) and anal intercourse. Partners usually have equal and interchangeable roles, contrary to popular belief concerning the 'female passive' partner and the 'active male' partner. A person can be more active in one relationship or more passive in another depending on circumstances, for example, the ages of the partners.

Women homosexuals practise mutual masturbation, oral sex (cunnilingus) and coital imitations with the use of a dildo (artificial penis).

THE PROBLEMS OF HOMOSEXUALS

The problems of homosexuals are largely caused by society's attitudes which are reflected by the family and then internalised by the homosexual himself.

Society portrays the homosexual at best as a figure of

ridicule, at worst as a target of verbal and physical abuse. Homosexuals are regarded with loathing and disgust, particularly by men. The homosexual who acknowledges that he is one may internalise these views and be full of self-loathing and disgust, and may well dress and behave in the stereotyped ways expected of him. Why are men in particular so antagonistic to homosexuality? The antagonism usually hides fears and anxiety. Homosexuality is equated with femininity which means weakness and submissiveness, whereas masculinity is equated with strength, toughness and aggression. The more insecure a man is about his self-image the more will he be anxious to guard it against any threat, real or imagined. The homosexual constitutes such a threat since he is seen as an example of what the man might become, and so he must be attacked. The young men who go in for 'queer bashing' do so because they are uncertain about their masculinity.

Given these attitudes it is hardly surprising that the man who suspects that he might be homosexual either vehemently denies it to himself or others or if he does acknowledge himself to be one then he is careful not to let anyone but his own homosexual friends know about it. He is forced to lead a life of secrecy. His loving and sexual relationships cannot be admitted. As a result, these relationships cannot develop and evolve as heterosexual ones do and hence are more likely to break down. This probably accounts for the homosexual's reputation for promiscuity.

The fear of being homosexual probably also leads many to marry in the hope of being 'cured'. These marriages are often under constant stress and threat of breakdown.

It is against this background that the Gay Liberation Movement must be seen. For an account of its rise and development see Altman (1974). The Gay Liberation Movement urged homosexuals to 'come out', to be 'blatant not latent', that is to acknowledge their homosexuality publicly. This also meant self-acceptance as worthwhile and equal human beings. 'Gay' was used to mean a 'celebration' of homosexuality.

There are several areas of difficulty for which the homosexual may seek help in relation to his homosexuality. Before dealing with these it must be remembered that homosexuals, like others, may need help with housing, work, money and also when a relationship ends or a loved one dies. These problems may have little or nothing to do with the homosexuality *per se*. Thus the social worker will need to guard against attributing any or all of the individual's problems to his homosexuality. Similarly the homosexual, like the heterosexual, can experience problems with sexual dysfunctions such as impotence or premature ejaculation which again are not caused by the homosexuality itself. Referral for psychosexual counselling and/or modified Masters & Johnson therapy may be appropriate for these cases, as with the heterosexual (Masters & Johnson 1979).

Problems to do with homosexuality itself may be concerned with the following:

1) Loneliness and the difficulty of meeting other homosexuals.

2) *Self-acceptance and conflict about sexual orientation:* The individual may acknowledge his sexual attraction to the same sex but despise himself for it. He may be a married man with children who got married in order to 'cure' his homosexual desires. Every once in a while the attraction becomes too great and so contact is made with homosexuals, sometimes in public lavatories. Fearing exposure and involvement with the law and the possible break-up of his marriage, he presents for help. The request may be to change his sexual orientation so as to be fully heterosexual. Although early learning experiences may determine the development of homosexuality, any attempt to 'unlearn' it by means of treatment, whether psychotherapeutic or behavioural, has met with limited success. The success rate for both methods is about 40 per cent (Bancroft 1974). Success is dependent on a number of factors:

1. Why the person wishes to change. If this is due to society's attitudes, referral by courts or pressure from relatives or guilt and depression associated with the break-up of a relationship, success is unlikely.

2. Whether the person has had heterosexual as well as homosexual relationships. If the relationships are exclusively homosexual, success again is unlikely.

3. The extent to which the person regards himself as homosexual. Should he feel that homosexuality is alien to him, then the chance of change is said to be improved. However, this feeling may be more the result of strong denial of homosexuality.

4. The extent to which his masturbating fantasies are homosexual or heterosexual. Again, if these are exclusively homosexual, change will be difficult to effect.

5. The person's age. A person over thirty-five is unlikely to change his sexual orientation.

TREATMENTS AVAILABLE

The treatments available to attempt to change sexual orientation are individual psychotherapy and behaviour therapy. Referral to a psychiatrist via the general practitioner is usually necessary. Until recently the main behavioural therapy offered was aversion therapy, which involved giving small electric shocks in association with homosexual fantasies. Since the results were disappointing (not to mention the moral dilemma associated with such unpleasant treatment) this form of treatment is rarely used. More attention is now paid to facilitating heterosexual interest by modifying masturbation fantasies in a heterosexual direction. An attempt is also made to improve social skills and help is given using role play with female volunteers on how to approach a woman and how to initiate conversations. A limited trial period is usually agreed upon with specific goals, and further treatment only takes place if some progress has been made. Fewer requests are now made to change sexual orientation. Help with acceptance of homosexuality and overcoming loneliness can be provided by direct referral by the social worker or self-referral to one of the counselling homosexual organisations such as Friend or the Albany Trust (for addresses, see p. 323). These organisations exist to befriend, support and counsel homosexuals. They also provide opportunities for homosexuals to meet socially.

Marital therapy, from either a marriage guidance counsellor or a psychosexual counsellor, may be appropriate where the man is married but finds that his homosexual interest is interfering with his marriage. Sometimes the wife will present for help when she discovers her husband's homosexual involvement. There may also be a concomitant sexual problem in the marriage such as premature ejaculation or lack of response on the part of the wife. Women married to homosexual men sometimes react very strongly on discovery of the homosexuality. They feel rejected (as happens if the husband is having an affair with a woman), but they also feel they cannot compete. Remarks such as 'If it was a woman I'd know what to do' or 'I just can't see what he fancies in another man' are commonplace from women who discover that their husbands are having a homosexual relationship. If they are uncertain about their own sexual attractiveness, then the situation is much worse. Divorce may be seen as the only answer, especially if the man feels he cannot or does not want to change. Where he does,

referral for psychotherapy or behavioural therapy is indicated.
Occasionally homosexual feelings suspected when dealing with a marital problem are vehemently denied. Referral to a homosexual agency may be too threatening and may precipitate a breakdown. Referral to a psychotherapist may be necessary.

HOMOSEXUALITY AND THE ADOLESCENT

Homosexual relationships or attachments can be a phase of adolescence. It is difficult to predict whether an adolescent will definitely be exclusively homosexual. The pattern of repeated homosexual relationships is usually seen retrospectively with no interest or emotional involvement with the opposite sex continuing through life. Thus if an adolescent presents with the fear of being or becoming a homosexual he cannot be given a definite answer about it. His fear and anxieties need to be explored. He may well be shy and timid with the opposite sex and have failed to make a long-lasting relationship and therefore fears he may be homosexual even where he has no sexual interest in his own sex. He will need help in making relationships, doing role play in a one-to-one situation where the social worker may help the young person learn social skills, what to say and how to say it when meeting a girl/boy for the first time. The social worker can introduce the young person to a club or disco.

Where the young person does appear fixed in his homosexual orientations, the social worker must accept the right of each individual to make his own sexual choices. The young person may still need help with problems of sexual relationships.

Mention has been made earlier that, in the opinion of one writer (Hertoft 1976), young people often have homosexual advances made to them and the majority learn how to deal with them. However, some young people may need help to cope with unwanted advances, whether homosexual or heterosexual.

Furthermore, social workers will have in their care vulnerable adolescents who because of earlier deprivation and/or bad parenting may be at risk from seduction by an apparently caring older teenager or adult. There is a risk that such an adolescent may be exploited and the seduction, whether of a homosexual or heterosexual nature, may be the prelude to prostitution, though it may not determine once and for all their sexual orientation. Such adolescents need careful and consistent handling by the same worker over a prolonged period of time. How adolescent girls use and abuse their sexuality will be considered in Chapter 13. The families and parents of homosexuals need help to deal with their feelings regarding homosexuality so that they can accept the homosexual as a person. The knowledge that their son is homosexual can be traumatic. It occasions much self-blame. In extreme cases the son may be rejected altogether and forced to leave home. The parents should be informed that the cause of homosexuality is largely unknown and that they are in no way to blame for their son's homosexuality. Attempts should be made to impress upon the parents that their son, apart from his sexual orientation, is exactly like other people. Referral to Parents Enquiry (an organisation founded to help the parents of homosexuals, and homosexuals themselves can be helpful.

FEMALE HOMOSEXUALITY

Female homosexuals rarely present themselves for treatment *per se* for their homosexuality, though they may seek help when a relationship breaks up or a loved one dies.

Problems are now being presented, however, where the charge of lesbianism may prevent a woman getting custody of her children in a divorce case. There is no evidence that children are damaged by being reared in a lesbian household.

DENIAL OF HOMOSEXUALITY

Mr and Mrs A., a young, attractive, rather boyish couple in their late twenties, were referred to a psychosexual clinic by a psychiatrist. Mrs A. had been under treatment for insomnia, depression and agoraphobia. She had no interest in or enjoyment from, sex. She gave a history of a loveless childhood and had begun to have sex early in her teens, looking for excitement, but had never enjoyed intercourse. Mr A. cheerfully admitted he had had occasional 'blow-outs' in public lavatories when men would practise fellatio on him. He found this wildly exciting. He denied that his blow-outs were homosexual, or that he was homosexual, since no feelings were attached. He had been drawn to his wife since she accepted his 'blow-outs'. Sex between them was infrequent. He gave a history of a seductive

and thrice married mother. He sometimes overheard his mother
having intercourse when in his teens and became excited and
would masturbate. Women were idealised and sex with his wife
had to be in the male superior position. He could not let her 'go
down there', i.e. touch his penis with hand or mouth, and he
did not like to touch her. For him love and sex were almost
completely divorced: he loved his wife but did not want sex
with her; he wanted sex with men but could not love them.
When the doctor attempted to explore this separation between
love and sex, treatment was broken off. Thus even the possibility of homosexual feelings had to be denied since this aroused
extremely anxious and painful feelings which threatened both
the self-esteem of the man and the marriage. In marrying his
wife he married someone who was not threatening or demanding sexually. Marriage also provided a safe cover of respectabil-
ity from which he could continue his homosexual experiences
and a facade that he was really a 'normal' man. He was very
much at risk of being caught and prosecuted.

5

Sexual Variations

What has been regarded as normal (and, therefore, acceptable and permissible) sexual behaviour has varied widely among different cultures and at different times. In Western society under Christian influence it has been customary to regard any form of sexual behaviour other than straightforward heterosexual intercourse (penis in the vagina) as deviant or perverted and in some cases unlawful. The importance of reproductive sex was stressed. Thus oral sex, anal intercourse, masturbation and homosexuality have all at times been regarded as perversions (and still are by some) since they do not lead to the creation of life. As perversions they were put alongside rape, paedophilia and bestiality. Absurd anomalies exist in the law with regard to sexual offences as a result of this emphasis on reproductive sex. Anal intercourse, since 1967 no longer regarded as a criminal activity between consenting males over twenty-one, is still a punishable offence between husband and wife whether the wife consents or not. It is questionable whether what two consenting adults do sexually, even if this is regarded by others as perverse or immature, should be a matter for the law. It is perhaps a question of good sexual manners. Should one partner find a particular aspect of sex, e.g. oral sex, distasteful, then this may, where it causes distress, require psychosexual counselling.

Chesser (1971) suggested a new dividing line in sexual behaviour between those acts done with mutual consent (social) and those done against another's will (anti-social). The former included sexual intercourse, mutual masturbation, oral sex, homosexuality, flagellation, fetishism, transvestism and oral intercourse; the latter exhibitionism, voyeurism, indecent assault, rape and offences against children. It should be noted that only one act in the social group is illegal, namely anal intercourse between a man and a woman. All the acts in the anti-social group are also sexual offences punishable by law, and rightly so, as they involve exploitation and possible violence to the other person. Chesser's classification will be used here, though offences against children will be looked at separately in Chapter 7, 'Paedophilia and Incest' — though, of course, not all incest involves children. Apart from oral sex, mutual masturbation and female homosexuality, all of the remaining acts are carried out by men. This may be due to the enormous anxiety which surrounds potency and the ability to sustain an erection. Having an erection (as stated earlier) is not a willed process under conscious control (although some Indian gurus claim the opposite). Sexual variations are not mutually exclusive but may be found combined in the same person.

CAUSES OF SEXUAL VARIATIONS

The causes of sexual variations are not known for certain at present, though various psychological explanations have been put forward. These will be looked at in more detail under each variation, though some general points will be made here. Men who manifest sexual variations tend to feel sexually unattractive and inferior and hence avoid sexual competition. This is far from the popular view that they are sexually very potent and filled with insatiable desire. In fact such men, believing themselves undesirable, often have great difficulty in making or sustaining sexual and loving relationships and may have to turn to prostitutes for sexual satisfaction. Sexual variations are manifested in varying degrees of intensity and are often compulsive and repetitive. They tend to be associated with much fantasising and sexual daydreaming of a bizarre nature. The variations may be exacerbated by stress in other areas of the individual's life; for example, marital difficulties or job pressure.

Storr (1964) sees the variations as resulting from deep feelings of sexual guilt and inferiority which have persisted from childhood. These feelings have their origin in strict negative parental views on sex and either extreme parental possessiveness (not allowing the child to grow up) or parental rejection. The parents also fail to form adequate models of masculinity or femininity for the child. As not all children growing up in such homes manifest sexual variations in later life, it is also postulated that those individuals who do must be especially susceptible in some way, by being very sensitive or impressionable. There is no evidence that men who manifest these variations are less intelligent than others.

Before leaving the causes, the negative influence of advertising on ideas of sexuality should be stressed. Advertisers display men and women who are not only very attractive sexually but also radiate extreme sexual self-confidence. This can be intimidating for people who are reasonably comfortable with their sexuality. How much more damaging it must be for those who are uncertain about their sexual attractiveness! The implication of such sexual images is that only those with similar looks can find a sexual partner and have an enjoyable sex life.

TREATMENT OF SEXUAL VARIATIONS

Various kinds of treatment are available through the National Health Service, private practice or voluntary bodies. The treatments include individual psychotherapy, psychosexual counselling, marital counselling, behavioural therapy and drugs. However, the results of treatment are disappointing, mainly because the man himself rarely presents for treatment unless he is in conflict with the law. Since his behaviour provides some satisfaction, it does not seem a problem to him and he is reluctant to give it up. It is often the sexual partner, usually the wife, who presents for help as she may recently have discovered the behaviour or can no longer tolerate it or is fearful of its effects on the children (particularly teenage) of the marriage. Where the wife does present, an attempt should be made to involve the husband. The marriage, its strength and weaknesses, and what the couple mean to each other can then be explored with a view to effecting some sort of compromise over the sexual behaviour which is tolerable to both. To accomplish this, however, implies that the couple really do care for each other and want the marriage to continue.

Behaviour therapy

Different forms of behaviour therapy have been tried, but with limited success. Since the variation is regarded as resulting from childhood conditioning or faulty learning, the aim is to alter the conditioned response. The behavioural approach is time-consuming and is spread over the course of a year. The methods used can be divided into 'positive', aimed at increasing normal behaviour, and 'negative', aimed at removing variant behaviour. For a detailed exploration of what is offered see Bancroft

(1974). The positive approach is used first to lessen the anxiety involved in sexual contacts and then to increase sexual responsiveness. This is done by means of relaxation technique combined with imaginary situations that the person finds alarming. The less alarming situations are imagined first, and once comfort is achieved the more frightening ones are dealt with. Where the techniques fail, 'aversion' therapy may be used. This is the 'negative' approach. It is hoped that by inducing a distaste for the object or person that has become sexually exciting the behaviour will be controlled or given up. This is done by associating the object with an unpleasant experience such as an electric shock. Aversion therapy has claimed some success with transvestism and fetishism. However, the aversion techniques are somewhat less successful than other behavioural approaches (Bancroft 1976).

Behaviour therapy and individual psychotherapy are available from some psychiatric departments; referral by the general practitioner is usually necessary. Counselling of the couple or one of the partners is available from marriage guidance and psychosexual counsellors' clinics. Referral by the social worker or self-referral is usually acceptable.

Drug treatment

There is considerable controversy about using drugs in the treatment of sexual variations as this has been seen as being less in the interest of the person and more in the interest of society. Also, unfortunately, the drugs used to decrease male sexual drive (female hormones) have serious side effects. A new drug that has been used to reduce sexual drive, cyproterone acetate, seems to produce less side effects though its use requires further investigation (Bancroft 1974). Its effects on sexual function may take several months to wear off. It must be reiterated that drugs alter sexual drive but not sexual orientation.

SOCIAL ACTS

Sadomasochism

Only the milder forms are included here. The brutal sadist who may commit murder and who may be a rapist or paedophile is dealt with later. Fortunately such people are rare.

Sexual excitement is obtained from the infliction of pain (sadism) or from the reception of it (masochism). The two may coexist in the same person. Hardcore pornography consists largely of sadomasochistic acts. There are degrees of sadomasochistic behaviour from the infliction of mildly painful stimuli to beatings (flagellation). Minor sadomasochistic rituals such as teasing are part of the normal sexual arousal for many couples. Whipping, biting, slapping are typical acts of physical pain inflicted by the sadist. Sarcastic remarks are another form of sadistic behaviour.

Sadism gets its name from the Marquis de Sade, a French writer who derived sexual pleasure from inflicting pain on women and spent many years in prison; masochism from an Austrian cavalry officer, Sacher-Masoch. He had a desire to be humiliated and punished by women.

Sadomasochism is found mainly among men, though there are women who exhibit masochistic tendencies in wanting to be overcome before allowing intercourse to take place.

Both sadists and masochists find it difficult to obtain sexual satisfaction in an equal relationship. Both treat the sexual partner as extremely powerful. In the case of the sadist the partner has to be forced into submission. Sadistic behaviour relieves feelings of inferiority and reassures the sadist that he is more powerful than the partner. The masochist, on the other hand, needs to hand himself over to the partner. He can then regress to a childish state where he no longer has to make decisions or take responsibility. Thus the powerful partner by punishing him relieves him of his guilt and at the same time stimulates him sexually. The masochist can then feel free to abandon his control over his impulses and can 'let go' — be sexual and yet safe.

Sadists and masochists also want their partner to enjoy their part. This is difficult for the extreme sadomasochist who then has to resort to prostitutes who will simulate pleasure. Conversations with prostitutes reveal that a large number of their clients are sadomasochist. In ordinary life the sadomasochist is usually mild-mannered and unassertive.

Within marriage degrees of sadomasochism appear to be tolerated and may form part of the sex play that ends in intercourse. If the man's potency depends, for example, on being tied up as a preliminary to intercourse, the wife may be willing to participate. Problems may arise when the behaviour gets more extreme and results in beatings that cause injury or where the behaviour becomes a substitute for intercourse and the sexual needs of the woman are ignored.

The man addicted to masochistic practices may use pornographic material to masturbate in such a way as to threaten his own life; for example, partial self-strangulation. Death has resulted in some instances.

Treatment The problem may be presented by the woman who may find her husband's behaviour becoming even more extreme. Conjoint marital therapy, i.e. seeing both partners to effect some sort of compromise that will limit the husband's behaviour to a more acceptable level for the wife, for example by being verbally abusive rather than physically so, can be used. Behavioural modification, particularly of the aversive variety, is inappropriate as it may encourage sadomasochistic fantasies for the obvious reasons that the masochist will enjoy it!

Fetishism

This is seen in men. Erotic arousal is centred on an object or article of clothing. There are degrees of fetishism from the mild, fairly common, condition in which the fetish serves as the means by which the man ensures his potency to the extreme form where the fetish replaces the person and is used for masturbation. The fetish is usually quite specific. Articles of underwear, corsets, gloves, high-heeled shoes, rubber, leather and satin have a strong, unexplained, appeal for the fetishist. The fetish may be part of the body, hair, thighs, feet, ears and so on. This can be an intensification of the tendencies seen in most men. Thus some men 'go' for breasts, others for legs. Fashion is devoted to cultivating aspects of the female body in sequences. One year the emphasis is on breasts, another on thighs. Many female fashions tend to make women appear helpless and weak. This appeals to men since it allows them to feel superior and protective. (The young seem to be trying to escape this by the unisex fashion of jeans and tee shirt.) Most fetishists are heterosexual.

There is some disagreement among analysts as to what the fetish actually represents. Freud (1905) supposed that the fetishist is especially terrified of castration. He thus has to pretend that women really do possess penises. The fetish acts as a reassurance by representing the missing female penis. Freud (1905) also thought that the velvet and fur beloved by some fetishists represented female pubic hair. It could also be postulated that the fetish is used as a 'comforter' in childhood masturbatory practices. The attachment to a favourite blanket, for example, is well known in children deprived of maternal affection. On the other hand, perhaps being able to be erotically excited by one aspect of the mother (such as her clothing or feet) guards against forbidden incestuous involvement with the mother herself. Hadfield (1950) regards the fetish as a breast substitute — the first loved object of the infant before the mother herself. Storr (1964) sees the fetishist as suffering from intense sexual guilt and sexual inadequacy. This makes him feel anxious on every sexual occasion. He therefore relies on something (the fetish) which has served to arouse him in the past. Women may seem frightening to him and thus inhibit an erection. He may also fear castration by the vagina and so substitute something less alarming as a feminine symbol (the fetish) as the focus of sexual excitement. Many fetishists also manifest compulsive traits such as a tendency to hoard or obsessional cleanliness. Occasionally the desire for a fetish promotes stealing. Some fetishes are associated with sadomasochistic practices such as being trodden on by leather boots. Transvestism can be associated with a fetish about particular kinds of women's clothes. Sometimes a handicapped person may be a fetish for certain individuals.

The man may keep his fetish a secret and merely fantasise on the object. Problems may arise when he asks his wife to participate in his fantasies, such as wearing particular articles of clothing. The woman may fear he loves the object rather than her, or if such clothes make her look or feel ridiculous she may seek help. She may also seek help where the fetish becomes an obsession and the man withdraws from any sexual contact with her.

Treatment Marital therapy with the involvement of the husband to effect some sort of compromise which is tolerable to both. Behavioural 'aversion' therapy has claimed some success (Marks *et al.* 1970). Obviously for treatment to succeed the man must truly want help.

Some illustrative cases

Case 1 Mrs A turned up at a walk-in advice centre distraught. Her husband had a 'thing' about rubber. He would put on rubber pants, urinate into them and then masturbate. He used to do this in private but was now insisting on doing it in the marital bed. There had been no sexual contact between them for about six months. They had three small children who were causing anxiety at school because they were so quiet and withdrawn. Mr and Mrs A were referred to a psychosexual doctor. A family tree revealed that Mr A seemed to follow the family pattern of being an unloved boy. Girls were much loved and wanted. At his birth his mother was afraid to tell his father that she had had a son. Later a sister was born whom father adored. The family was very strict and religious. Mr A could trace his rubber fetish back to an occasion in his childhood when his sister wore a rubber cape (on which he dwelt lovingly in his description). He described a lonely and introverted childhood. Treatment was based on trying to effect a compromise situation between the couple, who cared for each other and did not want their marriage to break up. Mr A did not want to give up his fetish, so it was arranged that he would indulge it two nights a week when his wife was at evening class. Intercourse was resumed after time spent on mutual caressing. The couple were seen regularly over a year and progress was reasonably maintained. The children are now doing well at school. However, in times of stress Mr A reverts back to his former frequency. Mrs A is then tempted to leave home and has to be supported to stay.

Case 2 Carol was a small, pretty woman of about thirty, married but childless. She cried during her first interview almost the entire time. In between sobs she described her unhappy marriage of five years. Her husband insisted that she wore corsets all the time. He would then sneak up behind her and slip his fingers between the corset to her buttock. He would then masturbate. Intercourse was practically non-existent. Any suggestion from her that they should seek help was met with violence. She had been fat and unattractive when they first met. She had been flattered by his attentions and felt he loved her for herself. They had intercourse regularly before they married. After marriage her self-confidence grew. She lost weight and wore more attractive clothes and threw away the tight-fitting corsets that she once wore. That was when the trouble started. He abused her and accused her of going off with other men and told her that if they were to stay together she must wear corsets. She used to wear them at home to please him, but recently he began to demand that she wear them all the time with clothes of the 1950s. She felt foolish and could tolerate the situation no longer. After several interviews she decided she would leave her husband and start divorce proceedings.

Transvestism or cross-dressing

Some men get excitement and satisfaction, either emotional or sexual, from dressing in women's clothes. This inclination to dress up in women's clothes is laid down early in life. It appears from some case histories that the men were forced to wear girls' clothes as a small child either because the mother wanted a girl or as a punishment. Either way the experience was invested with excitement. Sometimes sexual excitement is derived from dressing in female clothes and then masturbating in front of a mirror. Transvestism often has the element of a fetish about it in that particular kinds of garments are selected. There may also be sadomasochistic aspects with pleasure obtained from tight or restrictive clothing. Transvestites are usually heterosexual. Probably less than 1 per cent of the population are affected, though accurate figures are not obtainable as this is a secret activity. Transvestism may be manifested in childhood or after puberty. It can last throughout life. Some men get married in the hope of being cured.

Several explanations have been put forward to account for transvestism, though all the factors are not known for certain. The psychoanalytic explanation is that the transvestite fantasises that the woman possesses a penis and thus overcomes his castration anxiety; by putting on female clothes he identifies with this phallic woman. Havelock Ellis (1936) attributed transvestism to an exaggeration of the normal tendency to identify oneself with a beloved person. Storr (1964) sees the transvestite as achieving two aims. By dressing in female clothes and acting the role himself he can 'conjure up whatever kind of woman he likes'. He can then act the part he has always hoped a girl would act for him. Also, the transvestite 'becomes in phantasy the woman with whom in reality he has failed to make an adequately close relationship'. Benjamin (1967) sees transvestism and transsexualism (see below) as 'symptoms of the same underlying psychopathological condition; that of sex or gender role disorientation. Transvestism is the minor though more frequent; transsexualism the more serious though rarer disorder'. For the transvestite to fulfil his emotional needs, both a male and a female part are required. The male part on the whole predominates so that he can be husband and father, but the rewards of dressing up and pretending to be a female may be necessary for emotional tranquillity. Transvestites often talk in terms of 'emotional relief' or 'a sense of peace and release'. Unfortunately, this behaviour may also be accompanied by guilty feelings sparked off by the knowledge that it transgresses social codes.

Some men manage to hide their transvestism from their wives; others share it with them. The reaction of the wife can vary from acceptance that may include buying clothes, wigs, etc. for their husbands, to disgust. In the latter case she may seek help or want a divorce. The transvestite may come into conflict with the law if found dressed as a woman in a female toilet. He may be apprehended for a breach of the peace. If he is found in a male toilet dressed as a woman he may be suspected of soliciting.

There is no information available concerning the effect on children growing up in a home in which the father is a transvestite.

Treatment   Since cross-dressing is intensely satisfying for some transvestites, treatment is unlikely to be sought unless the future of the marriage is at stake or there is a threat of dismissal from work. Aversion therapy has claimed some success (Marks *et al.* 1970) where the man is motivated to change. Individual psychotherapy may be necessary to help the transvestite come to terms with his feelings. The Beaumont Society exists to help and support transvestites. Marital therapy can be tried where the wife is aware of the situation and is distressed by it but the couple wish to remain together.

Transsexualism

This should be distinguished from transvestism, though the social worker is unlikely to meet a case. It means the incompatibility of an individual's anatomy with his psychological sexual identity. The vast majority of transsexuals are male. They have the genetic and anatomical characteristics of the male sex but reject maleness and wish to lead the life of women, emotionally, physically and sexually. Their need is often so desperate that they go from one doctor to another to effect the sex-change. The cause of transsexuality is postulated to lie in a mother-son relationship that is intense and close and excludes the other members of the family (Green R. 1969).

There are a few specialist centres in Britain and the United States that will perform these operations; about 2,000 people in the US have undergone them. Centres usually set conditions for the transsexual before they agree to operate, namely, that the individual must live as a member of the opposite sex for about two years and has undergone hormonal treatment. This needs to be given for 1–2 years prior to operation. A five-year follow-up study on 93 post-operative transsexuals showed that two-thirds of patients felt happier (Lamb 1975).

The incidence of transsexualism is not known, but may be 2 in 100,000 men and 1 in 400,000 women.

Anal intercourse

Sometimes known as the Italian form of birth control. This is a punishable offence (life imprisonment) in heterosexual relationships, which seems absurd as the act is not illegal between men over the age of twenty-one. Analytical theory postulates that the man who wishes to have anal intercourse is really a repressed homosexual. The incidence is unknown, as it is a private matter, though it is probably more widespread than is generally supposed. Anal intercourse is not harmful from the medical point of view, provided the anal sphincter is gently stretched before penetration. This is helped by using a lubricating jelly. It is advisable, however, *not* to insert the penis into the vagina after anal intercourse, since organisms may be transferred to the vagina, causing infection.

ANTI-SOCIAL ACTS

As stated earlier, these are also illegal. About 13,000 people are charged with 'sexual offences' in Britain each year; they form 0.5 per cent of all offences charged. 50 per cent of all sexual offences are charges of indecent exposure or soliciting (McGrath 1976). In 1972, 116 patients were in Broadmoor for having committed serious assaults of a heterosexual or homosexual nature (Hansard 1972).

Exhibitionism

This refers to the exposure of the genital organs, usually to strangers. It is a male disorder. While exhibiting himself the man may get an erection (though not always) and ejaculate. The man is usually heterosexual and may well marry. He is usually a weak, timid, insecure person, uncertain of his masculinity. He tends to have been brought up in a strict puritanical home and to have had limited sexual experience. Though he may be married, intercourse tends to be infrequent (Mathis 1969). The people exposed to are usually women or girls; in about half the cases they are under sixteen. The reaction the exhibitionist seeks is one of horror, fear and disgust. This gives him a sense of power and potency. Thus there are usually sadomasochistic aspects to such behaviour. The women are not usually molested. If the woman reacts hysterically it increases the man's sense of power. The best approach is for the woman to calmly ignore the act and suggest that the man should get medical help. Children and girls in particular should be informed about this behaviour and told what to do. It is then unlikely that the children will be afraid. The exhibitionist is rarely involved in serious crimes and is more a nuisance than a menace. For this reason, and as he is so often a sad, pathetic person, he is more to be pitied than blamed. In older men the behaviour can be precipitated by unhappiness at home, marital problems and stress at work.

Exhibitionism is the commonest of all sexual offences. There are about 3,000 convictions per year. Most offenders are charged once. About 20 per cent are charged again, usually within a short time. Indeed, some exhibitionists seem to have a compulsive need to get caught. These are the ones who exhibit themselves more than once in the same place. Of course, the element of danger involved in risking discovery may be a powerful sexual stimulant in itself.

Treatment Both psychodynamic and behavioural, mainly aversion therapy, has been tried with a measure of success (Routh 1971). If masochism is a strong element in the disturbance, the aversion therapy with its emphasis on punishment is likely to exacerbate the problem. Marital therapy may be necessary if the man is married. The wife's reaction to the knowledge that her husband is an exhibitionist is likely to be one of disgust. There is then a strong possibility that she will take divorce proceedings. The stress on the man may thereby increase, which is likely to exacerbate the exhibitionism. As already mentioned, there may already be pre-existing marital and sexual difficulties which have precipitated this behaviour in the first place.

Voyeurism

This refers to the 'Peeping Tom' who gets pleasure from watching other people's sexual activity or from watching women undressing. It is an offence. It occurs only in men. Like the exhibitionist, the voyeur is usually harmless and flees on discovery. Many voyeurs and exhibitionists feel they were rejected in childhood and do not feel sufficiently masculine. By exhibiting themselves and spying they feel a sense of power that bolsters their masculinity, and because there is no relationship involved they do not risk rejection.

Frotteurism

This refers to men who rub themselves up against women in crowded trains, for example. They may masturbate to orgasm.

Acceptance by a professional worker of the person who manifests these disorders, together with care and concern, may be the best therapy, since traditional solutions to these problems seem so rarely to succeed.

6
Rape

During recent years there has been increasing interest in and concern about rape. This began in the United States in conjunction with the growth of the Women's Movement.

In the past rape has tended to be seen either as a joke (lie back and enjoy it) or as a shameful (and therefore hidden) event, particularly on the part of the victim. There are even those who hold the view that a woman cannot be raped.

The legal definition of rape is as follows. A man commits rape if:

a) he has unlawful sexual intercourse with a woman without her consent by force, fear or fraud (Sexual Offences Act 1956); and

b) at that time he knows she does not consent to intercourse or he is reckless as to whether she consents to it (Sexual Offences Amendment Act 1976).

The 1976 Act gave the right of anonymity to raped women (although at the discretion of the judge) and a direction that the woman's past sexual history should not be referred to unless the judge considers it relevant to the case.

A 'man' refers to a male over fourteen years, irrespective of the degree of sexual maturity. A boy under 14 can be charged with indecent assault and with aiding in rape.

A woman cannot be raped in law by her husband even if force is used, since it is tacitly implied that she gave continuing consent at the marriage ceremony. If force is used this can be the basis for an action for assault or grounds for divorce on the basis of cruelty. If the husband and wife are judicially separated then the man can be accused of rape. Intercourse is always unlawful if the girl is under thirteen years. If the man believes himself married to a girl between thirteen and sixteen, he cannot be accused of rape. Penetration of the vagina by hand or the use of bottles and broom handles does not constitute rape; this would constitute grievous bodily harm. If there is valid consent on the woman's part, the charge of rape or indecent assault cannot hold. The law does not recognise the validity of consent given by a young or mentally handicapped person. What constitutes valid consent can be extremely difficult to determine since it is influenced by what society has considered as acceptable sexual behaviour on the part of men and women. Thus, society as a whole expects men to initiate sexual advances in response to certain cues (in dress, demeanour and speech) from women. Women, in turn, are expected to control the extent of these advances and to limit them if they wish. Once a certain point has been reached, however, men are considered to be in the grip of an uncontrollable sexual desire which, once fully aroused, must be fulfilled. Women are expected to be able to gauge the level of this sexual excitement and to control it by their behaviour. Thus women are expected to be the guardians of sexual morality. Should they be the initiators of a sexual advance, they are not considered to be 'nice' women. These societal expectations surrounding sexual behaviour have consequently led to a number of beliefs about rape that are often accepted as facts, namely:

a) nice girls do not get raped (since they only allow limited sexual advances);

b) women ask for rape (they 'lead' men on by the way they dress, walk and talk);

c) women enjoy rape (because they asked for it);

d) women deserve rape (because they encouraged the men);

e) you can't thread a moving needle (she must have been willing).

Thus if a woman gets raped she must have provoked it in some way either in her dress or manner or even by being alone on a dark night or accepting a lift. The demonstration of provocation is used as a defence of the accused man. There are obviously differences in the kinds of situation where rape occurs. Thus rape can more easily be seen as indefensible in time of war or where a woman is attacked by an unknown man. However, where the man is an acquaintance or friend it might be felt that some degree of responsibility rests with the woman, though it must be questionable, regardless of the woman's behaviour, whether she deserves to be raped. It is often thought that if a woman does not resist the rape she must have given her consent. However, women who are attacked may well be in such a state of shock that they cannot resist or they may well fear physical violence if they do. The man, of course, may threaten violence unless the woman complies. Another difficulty involves the use and effect of alcohol. The woman who consents while under the influence of alcohol may regret it when sober. Should this be regarded as true consent, especially if the man has plied the woman with alcohol?

Most of the statistical and sociological facts about rape come from the United States where this problem is a cause for increasing concern in the large cities and has been studied extensively. Readers are referred to the original source material. A few of the most salient facts are presented here:

1. women of all ages, races, social classes and life styles have been raped;

2. rape often involves beating and the use of sticks and knives; 83 per cent of the rapes in the United States involve physical force to some degree;

3. very few rapists are referred for psychiatric treatment (in 1975 1 in 5 convicted rapists were sentenced to psychiatric institutions in Britain);

4. according to the US Federal Commission on Crimes of Violence, only 4 per cent of reported rape involved any provocative behaviour by the women;

5. women are raped in any situation: at home, out walking, at work. This contradicts the belief that rape occurs only late at night and that the woman deserves rape because she was running a risk;

6. only 4 per cent of reported rapes out of 645 were considered unfounded;

7. of women confronted with a threat to their life or physical well-being, 55 per cent were submissive, 27 per cent resisted and 18 per cent fought (Amir 1971).

About 1,000 cases of rape are reported to the police in Britain every year. This is probably an underestimate of the actual number of rape cases that occur, for a variety of reasons:

a) society's attitudes and beliefs about rape are such that the woman may feel that she will not be believed and that the police will not be sympathetic;

b) self-blame — incorporating society's attitudes, the woman may believe that she must have behaved in such a way as to provoke an attack;

c) wish not to relive a bad experience (it may take many months for the case to come to court). Black women especially are unlikely to report rape, from fear of an unsympathetic response and a wish to protect the man who, they believe, will be victimised by white society.

THE EFFECTS OF RAPE

The woman who has been raped, particularly where threats or force have been used, is usually in a state of shock. This may express itself as hysteria, extreme agitation, or withdrawal and an apparent lack of feeling. She needs gentle handling and the opportunity to talk about the rape and all aspects of it, including her feelings about it and her behaviour at the time.

Since women who have been raped have also internalised society's attitudes, they are often caught in a psychological double bind. As nice girls do not get raped, they are not nice girls. Also they must somehow have provoked the attack. Thus there may be an obsessional concern in finding causes for the attack with repeated incrimination. 'What did I do?' 'Why did it happen to me?' There may also be a strong tendency to blame themselves and hold themselves responsible. There may be intense angry and bitter feelings (understandable) against the rapist. This may spill over to include all men. It may take many months for the woman to recover from the experience. Some women develop agoraphobia and do not want to go out alone. They may be unable to have sex with their regular partner, since this recapitulates the attack. Some women never recover from rape, particularly where violence has been used. It may prevent them from responding to normal sexual overtures and be the cause of psychosexual problems. (In connection with this, when the first rape crisis centre was opened in 1976 in London many of the women who contacted the centre had been raped many years before. The anger, pain and humiliation they felt was still very much in evidence. Most of these women had never previously discussed the experience but had tried, unsuccessfully, to forget it.)

The partners of women who have been raped may react in a violent way with a wish to take revenge. This may later be replaced by doubts as to whether the woman provoked the attack, especially if the man was an acquaintance. Allied to this may be curiosity about whether the woman enjoyed it. The rape may expose the weakness of the relationship and any sexual difficulties. The man has to be helped to understand that the rape was an act of violence and not sex.

The rape may also precipitate problems within the family, especially if the girl is a young teenager and lives at home. The parents may blame themselves and feel they did not protect their daughter properly. They may learn at this time that their daughter has been involved in a regular sexual relationship. If they disapprove they may blame their daughter for the rape occurring. Thus they will need help both with the rape and with accepting their daughter's sexuality.

HELPING THE RAPED

The social worker may be the first person contacted. The woman should be told *not* to clean herself or remove her clothes. (Often the first thing she wants to do is to rid herself of the experience in the literal physical sense.) The social worker should accompany the woman to the doctor where she can be examined. Her physical state will be needed as evidence, together with blood-stained or semen-stained clothing. Sperm may not always be detected despite sexual assault, since some rapists fail to ejaculate (Burgess & Holmstrom 1974; Groth & Burgess 1977). Examination shortly after the rape will fail to reveal bruises, since these may take hours to develop. Pregnancy and VD tests will also need to be performed. Abortion may be necessary. If the woman wishes to report the incident to the police, the social worker should accompany her.

Since the rape may adversely affect the partner and family of the woman, these too may need help to talk about their feelings and attitudes towards it. Sexual relations should not be resumed until the woman wishes it. This, of course, may put a strain on the relationship. The man may feel rejected. He may then, if he is insecure about his sexuality, convince himself that the rapist was better at sex. Thus both the woman and the couple may need to be seen regularly for several months after the rape.

A Rape Crisis Centre, the first of its kind in Britain, was opened in London in 1976 with the purpose of providing 'legal, medical and emotional counselling by having a 24 hour phone service' (Rape Crisis Centre: First Report 1977). It also aimed to do research into the pattern and incidence of rape. The Centre was (and is) run by a group of women counsellors selected and trained by the Centre, most of whom work voluntarily. The Centre has medical and legal advisers. Women can contact the Centre directly. Anxiety is sometimes expressed that the existence of such centres (four other centres have subsequently opened — see list of Useful Addresses) will encourage rape. That is possible; however, it would seem more likely that such centres, carefully run, will lead to greater knowledge of rape and its effects, which might otherwise be concealed. Women are more likely to talk freely of their experience when they do not fear judgement or censure. Work done in Rape Crisis Centres in the United States suggests that women seem to recover more quickly from the effects of rape when they can discuss it with other victims and identify with each other.

ILLUSTRATIVE CASES

Case 1 Sarah was a 21-year-old student. She returned home late one evening in her parents' car. The lock-up garage was a short distance from her home. While she was putting the car away a young man attacked from behind and held a knife to her throat. He threatened to kill her and then raped her. He then ran off. Sarah reported the matter to the police who were helpful. Five women had been raped in the same vicinity by a man answering the description of Sarah's attacker. When he was finally caught it emerged that he had already served a prison sentence for rape. Sarah was on tranquillisers and could not go out alone for many months afterwards. She developed a tremor that took some time to clear up. Fortunately her boyfriend stayed with her and supported her.

Case 2: a past attempt at rape causing later psychosexual problems Julie, a married woman of thirty-four with four children, was referred for psychosexual counselling by the psychiatrist who was treating her for anxiety and depression. She had never enjoyed sex and now that the fear of pregnancy had been removed by sterilisation she had no excuse to refuse sex. She loved her husband and was fearful of losing him, hence the anxiety and depression.

During the first interview, during which there were many hesitations and pauses, she revealed that a man at work had attempted to rape her when she was sixteen. Julie knew little about sex (her parents were too embarrassed to discuss it). Recently, she had recurring nightmares of the man's face, 'all red and peculiar', above her and then of herself running. When she had tried to tell her parents what had happened, mother said she had too many other worries and though father said he would fix the man he did nothing. Julie was left to try and cope on her own. She expressed surprise at herself several times during the interview for talking about the incident. She had never told anyone else except her husband and even then not the details. It took several interviews for Julie to come to terms with what had happened. She needed to relive the experience and the feelings of helplessness and rage with both her attacker and her parents. After this some simple behavioural techniques (modified from Masters & Johnson) involving both Julie and her husband with emphasis on mutual caressing and permission to enjoy sex led to complete recovery. Julie was fortunate in that she had a loving and supportive husband.

THE RAPIST

Sociological studies of the kind done in America need to be done in England. At present the rape crisis centres are keeping careful records of the women who contact them. Information is also needed on the rapist, if only because most men are rightly angered by the idea held by the more extreme feminist groups that all men are potential rapists.

As few rapists are referred for psychiatric treatment this might imply that they do not have psychological problems. Convicted rapists tend to be of below-average intelligence, and to come from broken homes with weak, often alcoholic fathers and disturbed relationships with both parents. Two main types of convicted rapists have been described, the second more common than the first (Gebhard *et al.* 1965).

a) men who feel hostile towards women with strong sado-masochistic fantasies;

b) men with psychopathic personalities, who have little self-control and no remorse for the pain inflicted by them on others.

The act of rape defends against anxiety (about potency), and satisfies wishes to hurt and control (Groth *et al.* 1977). Thus rapists tend to have feelings of fear, contempt and hostility towards women. The London Rape Crisis Centre has found that rapists tend to be young (16 − 25 years). Rape may possibly cease (apart from those cases perpetrated by men with psychopathic personalities) when women are really seen to be equal to men and respected as such. This would refer to all women, not the exaggerated respect and cherishing reserved for some. 'Gang bangs', or rape by a group, usually of young men, appear to be carried out by those who need to impress their peers and have extreme anxieties about potency. There may also be an associated homosexual component − one group who raped a girl claimed when interviewed that it was 'doing it with your mates' that really counted.

Occasionally, of course, some women may allege that they have been raped to extricate themselves from the consequences of having sex, e.g. the teenage girl who finds she is pregnant and is fearful of parental reaction or the woman who feels that her request for abortion will be the more readily acceded to. The woman who has been rejected by her partner or is angry with him may claim that she has been raped. It is unfortunate that it is these cases which are used to discredit the real victims of rape.

7

Paedophilia and Incest

PAEDOPHILIA

Literally, paedophilia means the love of children. The man desires erotic pleasure from contact with a child, either by exposing himself, touching their genitals and/or getting them to touch his, or attempting penetration. The child, who can be male or female, is usually prepubertal, 6 − 11 years. Although the paedophile is portrayed as a dangerous sex maniac, violence in fact occurs in only a small minority of cases, though these are the ones that hit newspaper headlines. Kinsey *et al.* (1953) found that 20−25 per cent of his middle-class female sample had been directly approached when they were between four and thirteen years by adult males who attempted to make sexual contact. Studies show that the paedophile in the majority of cases is much more likely to be a friend or relative of the family or known to the child in some way such as a school caretaker rather than a complete stranger. This can be more damaging because the child is then uncertain whom to trust and who will believe him. The typical stereotype of the paedophile is that he is either an old man or mentally retarded. Work from the United States in particular suggests that this is not so. The majority of offenders commit their first offence before the age of forty and only a tiny proportion are psychotic or insane (Burgess *et al.* 1978). The child offenders are typically hetero and not homosexual.

Paedophiles have been divided into two main groups (Burgess *et al.* 1978).

(1) The *fixated* paedophile who has been primarily attracted to younger people from adolescence. Sexual relationships with adults tend to be avoided for fear of rejection and from feelings of inadequacy or inferiority. These offences are chronic and persistent. There are no feelings of guilt, shame or remorse and the sexual desires are experienced as compulsive.

(2) The *regressed* paedophile, who originally preferred adult

partners for sexual gratification. He often feels inadequate in the face of adult responsibilities and if the stress in his life is too great, for example with his marriage or job, he turns to a child for comfort. He is usually distressed and ashamed by his behaviour. At the time of the sexual activity he is usually depressed and does not think about what he is doing. Since the man usually is ashamed, treatment is easier and the progress better. Treatment for the fixated paedophile is more difficult.

It is often popularly supposed that force is always used in cases of paedophilia. However, in the majority of cases the adult wants an emotional relationship with the child and so bribery is used. It is only when this fails that the threat of physical force may be used, not with the intention of hurting the child, but in order to have sex. A small group of paedophiles (and these are the ones who gain the most publicity) gain pleasure from hurting the child. Thus the physical abuse and degradation of the child are essential for sexual excitement and gratification. This behaviour is usually premeditated.

For the fixated paedophile inept at social relationships, isolated and lonely, the child is easier to impress and overcome. With his deep-seated feelings of inadequacy, poor impulse control concerned with his own needs, and inability to tolerate frustration, the paedophile has been described as a 'psychological child in the physical guise of an adult' (Burgess *et al.* 1978). The paedophile may give a history of sexual abuse/incest as a child. It is possible that the child with whom the paedophile tries to make a relationship is in fantasy himself and that the love he gives to the child is what he himself would like to have received.

The law

It is always unlawful to have intercourse with a girl under the age of thirteen. Intercourse with a girl between thirteen and sixteen may not be unlawful in the following circumstances:

    a) the man believes her to be his wife;
    b) the man is below the age of twenty-four;
    c) the man has not been charged with a similar offence;
    d) the man has reasonable cause to believe that the girl by reason of her appearance and demeanour was over sixteen.

The Indecency with Children Act 1960 provides penalties for a man inviting children of either sex below the age of fourteen to touch or masturbate him with or without threats or force. If the man directly interferes with the child he can be charged with indecent assault. A homosexual offence takes place when one or both male partners is below the age of twenty-one.

Treatment

For the violent paedophile institutional care is necessary to protect children. For the 'regressed' paedophile psychiatric and/or social work help is needed to aid him through the crisis which led to the behaviour. For the fixated paedophile who is not violent there may be no alternative to institutional care or prison since these offences are persistent. This is unfortunate, not only because this increases the dependency these men already feel but because they may become the victims of physical abuse from other inmates. Hormone therapy on a regular basis to reduce sex drive (though not orientation) offers another possible approach.

Management of the child

A medical examination (provided the parent or guardian consents) should be performed whenever sexual abuse has occurred, whether recently or not. Children react in a variety of ways to sexual abuse. Much depends on the number of incidents, how long the child has been involved, whether violence has been used and the degree of shame and guilt felt by the child. The child may tolerate the situation for the affection received. This occurs particularly where the children are emotionally deprived. Ingram (1979) in a small study of 92 cases of sexual contact between adult and child found that in only six families could both parents be considered satisfactory. The paedophiles who are fixated on children sometimes claim that the children were seductive or provocative. This may possibly be true for those children who are rejected at home and who are searching for love. However, the children should not be held responsible for the behaviour of the adults concerned.

The child may react with indifference or denial or act out his distress in behavioural problems (eating, sleeping disturbances, bet wetting, school phobia or agoraphobia). The effect on the parents is variable. Some parents react with disgust and horror and self-blame, others are angry with the child. The parents' sexual relationship may be affected as also their physical health.

Work may suffer. Many parents take the view that the less the child talks about the assault the better, and so discourage discussion. It is important to help them realise that the more the child (and they) can talk about the experience the quicker he will recover. The child should be encouraged to lead his usual life as soon as possible, while the parents should be encouraged to support the child but not be over-protective and fearful. Of course, if the child does feel rejected and unloved at home, work will have to be done with the whole family, or with the mother and child if the former is not possible. It should be remembered that, provided violence has not been used, sexual assaults by a stranger or acquaintance are far less traumatic for the child than similar assaults by a relative or parent. The parental response is significant here. If the parents over-react and become hysterical this can have a more damaging effect than the attack itself.

INCEST

Incest refers to sexual acts and/or intercourse which take place between two closely related people who cannot legally be married. The most common forms of incest are father/daughter, stepfather/stepdaughter, brother/sister, uncle/niece. Mother/son incest appears to be rare. Brother/sister incest is possibly the commonest form; it is perhaps less likely to come to the attention of the authorities, particularly when the brother and sister are of comparable ages.

Incest is an almost universal taboo, although certain kinds of incestuous relationships have been permitted in some societies, e.g. brother/sister marriage in the royal families of the ancient Egyptians. It is not known what prompted the taboos and prohibitions that surround incest, whether it was due to a desire to preserve family unity and prevent sexual jealousy within the family, to encourage mating outside the family circle circle, to protect the children or for healthy psychosexual development of the child (Maisch 1973).

It is difficult, for obvious reasons, to obtain statistics for incest, though it is probably far more prevalent than is admitted. About 200–300 cases are reported to the police each year and there are about 100 convictions. Although it is supposed to be more prevalent in isolated rural areas, there is little statistical evidence to support this.

The law

Until the nineteenth century incest was punishable by the ecclesiastical courts. In the later nineteenth century, cases of incest were not infrequently presented as rape. Several unsuccessful attempts were made between 1893 and 1908 to establish incest as a criminal offence. They were resisted on the grounds that incest was rare. There was also a fear that there would be an increase in cases if incest was advertised by having a special law. However, in 1908 incest was made a criminal offence, possibly as a result of a change in the Home Office view. The 1956 Sexual Offences Act now incorporates the law on incest. Section 10 provides that it is an offence for a man to have sexual intercourse with a woman whom he knows to be his granddaughter, daughter, sister, half-sister or mother. This applies whether or not the relationship is traced through lawful wedlock. The penalty is seven years' imprisonment, and two years' for attempted incest. If the girl is under thirteen, there may be imprisonment for life. Consent is no defence.

Psycho-social factors

Though incest occurs in families of all social classes, it is popularly supposed to occur in economically deprived families living is overcrowded accommodation and for the victims to be mentally subnormal. From the studies carried out so far it would appear that by far the most important factors are to do with faulty family relationships, particularly those between husband and wife and mother and daughter which precede incest. Thus incest is not the *cause* but the *result* of a disturbed family situation. In some families the husband appears to be looking more for a mother than a wife and while providing financial support does not provide emotional support. If the wife then becomes self-sufficient and independent she may reject the husband and react with indifference towards him. The husband then turns to the daughter as surrogate wife-mother, at first to attend to his physical needs such as cooking and washing his clothes, and later his sexual ones. In other instances the wife is too dependent on the husband, who, being overwhelmed by her emotional demands, turns to his daughter for attention (Burgess *et al.* 1978). Sometimes the father is authoritarian and strict (the family tyrant), socially controlling his wife and children (Maisch 1973). As with the paedophile, the man who commits incest often has poor impulse control and an inability to tolerate frustration, and has to gratify his needs immediately and without thought for the needs of others.

The mother is more often than not aware of the relationship but colludes either for fear of reprisal from the husband and loss of economic support or because it spares her from sexual relations with him. Indeed she may play an active role in transferring the responsibility for gratifying the father's sexual needs to a child in the family (Burgess *et al.* 1978), especially when she does not want or enjoy sex. According to Pincus & Dare (1978) the mother may get vicarious pleasure from the relationship as a result of her own incestuous fantasies. Thus her daughter is really herself receiving the kind of attention from father that she would have liked. The relationship between mother and daughter tends to be negative and is often hostile.

Physical ill health and pregnancy in the mother and her absence from home leaving the father alone with the children also seem to be contributory factors. Alcoholism, though not necessarily always present, does seem to play a part either as a solace for an unhappy marriage or in lessening self-control, or both. Overcrowding does not seem to be a significant factor in most cases and the girl is not invariably mentally retarded.

The common age for involvement in an incestuous relationship is 10–11 years for the girl. The girl is usually (though not invariably) the eldest daughter. The father may develop a sexual interest in the girl when he becomes aware of her sexual development, notably her breast development. Incest usually occurs at the time of the first period (Burgess *et al.* 1978) or shortly after. It tends to go on for a number of years. As the daughter grows older so the father may turn his attention to the younger girls. Occasionally, the father can be involved with several daughters at one time.

According to Maisch (1973) the girl is not sexually provocative but tends to accept the relationship in a passive and tolerant way. Cavallin (1966) found that 60 per cent of incest victims were voluntary participants. There are various reasons for this. (1) Children are in a weak position *vis-à-vis* adults and are expected to obey them even when the behaviour advocated is wrong. (2) The relationship between the adult and child is not always a negative one. There may be warmth and emotional dependence, especially where the mother is rejecting. (3) There are fears of reprisals, of not being believed, of being blamed and rejected. (4) The child may not have the words or understanding to describe to others what is happening. (5) The child may obtain material rewards and be favoured more than the other siblings. Sometimes the mother will have abandoned the home leaving the children with father. The father then turns to the oldest daughter who becomes both 'wife' and mother to the other children. Where the girl is already a teenager she may be unwilling to relinquish her role and the power it gives her.

What is the sexual involvement? Although it is often supposed to refer to actual intercourse, this may not occur. It may start with undressing the child, fondling of the sex organs, fingers in the vagina or rectum, oro-genital sex and ejaculation on the abdomen or between the legs. The child may be asked to masturbate the man. The sexual contact may proceed to full intercourse as the child gets older.

How is incest revealed? It has to be accepted that many cases may never come to the notice of the authorities. They may only be revealed in later life, for instance during psychosexual counselling. It may be suspected, but no definite proof may be obtained. A member of the family or one of the siblings may reveal it to the authorities. The girl herself may reveal it if she becomes pregnant or if the pressure to maintain secrecy is too great. She may not be able to complain directly but may manifest her distress by behavioural problems such as refusal to eat or sleep, staying away from school or running away from home. As the girl grows older and more sure of herself (through going to work and meeting people outside the family) she may disclose the relationship. The man in this situation often reacts by being extremely jealous and possessive, especially if there is a rival in the form of a boyfriend. The disclosure may then be an attempt to escape his control. Disclosure can also occur once the girl learns about society's views on incest. The guilt then experienced may be overwhelming. The girl may disclose that incest has taken place out of jealousy if father transfers his interest to another daughter. The first daughter may then behave more in the manner of a rejected lover than an abused daughter.

Effects of incest

These can vary enormously and depend on individual circumstances. Although outsiders may view the incestuous relationship with horror and disgust, it should not be forgotten that there may be positive aspects in the relationship for the child — the closeness, warmth and special attention, particularly if there are no other loving relationships. Thus incest may be less damaging than is commonly supposed. Sometimes the girl may enjoy the power and control she exerts over the father and the privileges she obtains as favourite. The degree of trauma seems to be greater the longer the relationship continues and the more incidents there are and also if there is much fear and shame. The need for secrecy, the broken trust and divided loyalty may be harder to endure than the sexual aspects. The distrust engendered may lead the girl to see relationships only in exploitative terms. She herself may use her sexuality to exploit others for money and material goods. Studies of prostitutes and drug addicts in the States have revealed a history of incest in a large number of cases. The girl may withdraw from adult relationships and be unable to be sexually responsive. Should she marry, she may fear telling her husband. The feelings of guilt, shame and anger, especially when the girl has had no opportunity to share them, may overshadow the rest of her life. Official discovery usually means the break-up of the family, with the father sent to prison, the mother suing for divorce and the children going into care. These may be more damaging than the effects of the incestuous relationship itself. The girl not only loses everything but may carry the blame and guilt for the break-up of the family.

The role of the social worker

The role of the social worker in the management of incest cases where the girl is under sixteen is similar in many respects to that of non-accidental injury (NAI). However, though most social service departments will have drawn up guidelines for dealing with NAI cases, it is unlikely that these will exist for incest cases. Further, back-up facilities with special expertise in this area may well not be available. In any suspected case of incest the social worker will need to discuss the management of it with his senior. The girl will need a full medical examination. A chaperone should be present.

In cases where incest is associated with violence, the social worker's role is clear. The child's welfare comes first, even if this necessitates removal of the child from the family. However, in cases where physical force is not used and where affectionate bonds do exist, there may be a reluctance to do anything that might jeopardise the child's position or the integrity of the family unit.

The social worker may suspect that incest is occurring. There may be behavioural problems, noted earlier. Any gonococcal infection in a child or foreign bodies inserted in the child's vagina or anus should lead to the suspicion of incest (Burgess *et al.* 1978). A complaint may be made by a relative or neighbour. Often those who make a complaint may wish to remain anonymous or refuse to substantiate their complaint when official action is proposed. If the mother makes the complaint the social worker's task will be easier since the child will have an ally in the family. Should the child complain, a direct confrontation between the child and the accused adult should be avoided unless separation of the child from the family can be ensured, since there is great risk of the child being intimidated (Burgess *et al.* 1978).

The decision whether or not to inform the police is a difficult one since this may lead to prosecution and the break-up of the family. Experience shows that once incest is known outside the family the chances are that it will cease. The threat of police action and the inevitable publicity should the case come to court may be sufficient to deter the father or stepfather from repeating the offence. However, intensive work (weekly or fortnightly visiting) will need to be done by the social worker, possibly in conjunction with a psychotherapist or psychiatric social worker from the local child guidance clinic or psychiatric department. The focus will be the parents' marriage and sexual relationship and the aim should be to strengthen both.

Special problems arise where the mother has abandoned the home and left the children with father and where the daughter involved is no longer a child. The father may lack confidence in making new relationships outside the family and may feel (with some justification) that no woman would want to take on the children as well. The daughter, as already stated, may enjoy her position — the fantasy of taking mother's place now a reality — so that she may be unwilling to give it up. She may be very much in need of the mother's love but her anger about being rejected may now cause her to take vindictive pleasure in replacing her. It may only be when the burdens of looking after the family outweigh the privileges that change is sought. The social worker may either have to decide to tolerate the incestuous relationship for a time to maintain family unity, particularly where there is evidence of care and affection, or break up the family and take the children into care. Setting aside the law, the girl will need to be faced with the fact that there can be little future in the relationship: that the roles of lover and father are opposing. Thus although many fathers may entertain fantasies of possessing their daughters, the majority do not act upon them. Indeed, one of the major tasks of parenthood is to let the child go freely to make its own life. It must also be impressed upon the daughter that the situation would not have arisen if the parents' marriage had been happier. It may be possible to arrange for a female relative to become more involved in the care of the children to free the daughter.

Case history A nineteen-year-old girl presented at the social service office with a complaint that her father was 'interfering' with her and that she thought she might be pregnant. During the interview she presented a confused picture. She insisted that she must get away while at the same time giving the impression that she enjoyed the situation. This was shown by the way in which she said how jealous her father was of her new boyfriend. It emerged that her father had been having intercourse with her regularly for four years. The daughter, along with four siblings, had spent considerable time in local authority care. The family were reunited when she was twelve. The relationship between mother and daughter had always been difficult and unhappy. According to the girl, her mother blamed her for the problems in her marriage. The mother had eventually abandoned the family (she had left and returned several times before) over a year earlier. Since then her daughter had assumed the mother's role and was caring for the younger children. The love and attention she was now receiving from her father was the only affection she had known. Pregnancy was confirmed, and at the girl's insistence the social worker made arrangements for the girl to go into a hostel. She stayed two days and then returned home. She miscarried soon afterwards and was heartbroken over the loss of the baby. She refused to allow the social worker to talk to her father and said she would deny everything if the police were involved. Her loyalty to her father and need of his love were such that she preferred this relationship with its sexual involvement rather than risk losing his love altogether, despite the fact that she knew it was illegal and condemned by society.

In California a unique (at present) programme for the treatment of incest cases has evolved since 1971. It is called the Child Sexual Abuse Treatment Programme (CSATP), and is described by Giarretto (in Burgess *et al.* 1978). The aim is to treat the man and his family without sending him to prison. It has been found that the authority of the criminal justice system is absolutely essential in treating incest (thus men are referred by the courts). The small number of drop-outs from treatment were those not involved with the police. There is close inter-action between the CSATP, the police, probation officers and the courts. The aims of the programme are threefold:

a) to maintain family integrity;

b) to teach people to assume personal responsibility for their actions;

c) to eliminate all incest in the family.

These aims are achieved by a combination of individual and group therapy. The decision whether to leave the child at home depends on whether the mother is against it, or abusive towards the daughter, and whether the daughter is passive and with-drawn, or the father has poor impulse control. Some of the guiding facets of the programme are that:

1. All the family must acknowledge, no matter how provocative or seductive the child, that the sole responsibility for the incest is the adult's. Thus the child must hear the mother say, 'You are not to blame. Daddy and I did not have a good marriage. That is why Daddy turned to you.'

2. The incestuous relationship is never condoned. The father must accept full responsibility. At the same time the hope is held out that the father will be able to maintain relationships with his family.

3. The girl needs to know that sexual feelings are good and normal.

Parents who have been treated have been helped to set up a Parents United self-help group led by co-therapists. The group gives support and helps the families develop social relationships. A similar group called Daughter United to support the victims has been started.

The results are promising. Over 600 families have been treated without relapse. The average age of the children affec-ted was 10–11 years and three-quarters of the cases were father-daughter incest. Fewer than 1 per cent were shown to be based on false allegations by the child. The families were white middle-class. Thus it is not known whether this approach would work with less articulate and poor families.

Giarretto has suggested that since not all workers can be trained to handle incest cases skilfully, local care teams com-prising a juvenile probation officer, a police officer, and a mental health worker should be set up.

Finally, the social worker may, of course, also be involved with adults whose sexual problems have their origins in early incest. These should be referred for psychosexual counselling. Where the woman refuses referral the social worker should provide her with the opportunity to talk about the incestuous relationship in detail and express her feelings of shame. Since there is much self-blame (as in rape cases), a statement that she cannot in any way be held responsible for its happening must be made.

Although father/daughter incest has been explored more fully here, since it potentially carries the most danger and is the form with which the social worker is more likely to be involved, the other forms should not be forgotten. There is probably less need for anxiety over brother/sister incest, especially when there is a small age difference, since there may be less opportunity for exploitation and violence. Similarly uncle/niece and grandfather/granddaughter incest may have fewer damaging effects since the contacts may be less frequent and the girl will be better able to avoid them. Obviously if the uncle or grandfather is living with the family there may be more difficulty. The situation may then share more of the features of father/daughter incest.

PART 2

Family Planning

8

Family Planning in Contemporary Society

With the recent changes in attitudes towards sex noted in the Introduction, it is perhaps strange to recall that family planning was once considered an inappropriate topic for polite conversation. With the anxieties surrounding over-population, the altered status of women, the emphasis on each child fulfilling his potential and the altered attitudes towards premarital sex, particularly among the young, sex, contraception and family planning are not only respectable subjects for discussion but almost mandatory. Thus everyone is expected to have views on these subjects, though often the views are based mostly on opinions rather than on a knowledge of the facts.

Although it often seems that birth control is a modern concept, most societies of the past did attempt to practise some form of birth control, either to limit the number of children, or to space children, or both. Thus the ancient Egyptians in 1800 BC advised sprinkling a gummy substance on the female genitals. Both abortion and infanticide have been used to control family size. The world's population was kept steady by high birth and death rates and high infant mortality rates. In the nineteenth century 150 babies died out of 1,000 live births in Britain. In 1977 the figure was 17.6. In the underdeveloped countries the number of babies dying is comparable to the figures for nineteenth-century Britain; a point to remember when dealing with families who have migrated to England.

During the nineteenth century both the death and birth rates began to decline and life expectancy began to increase. In 1850 the life expectancy for a baby girl at birth was 40 years, in 1900 it rose to 47 years and by 1976 it was about 70 years. The main reason for this is the control of infectious diseases, especially those which affect children. However, the mortality rate of children from disease in the western world is strongly related to social class, being higher in the lower socio-economic groups. Owing to the increase in life expectancy, a significant proportion of the population in Britain is over 60 years of age

(11 per cent in 1976). This compares with 3 per cent in the Indian sub-continent which has a preponderance of young people.

Since the mortality rate has been reduced, it is not necessary to produce a large number of children to ensure the survival of a few. In an advanced society, also, children are not needed as extra hands to work on the land or to act as an insurance against old age.

Alongside this smaller family size and contributing to it is the altered status of women, no longer confined or expected to be confined to the home and wholly concerned with motherhood. Two world wars hastened the emancipation of women from their homes. They were needed to do men's jobs working in factories making ammunition and they proved they could do it. Once the wars were ended women were not easily willing to forego the freedom and independence (particularly in having their own wage packet) they had known in order to return to the home. The advent of effective female methods of contraception (the cap in 1885, the IUD in the 1950s, the pill in the 1960s) and the rise and success of the birth control movement which was brought about mainly by women, consolidated their new-found freedom. Women now as never before had and have real control over their lives and options open to them denied in the past when repeated pregnancy was the inevitable consequence of being married.

At the same time the insight into individual development and psychology and the influence of the family on the individual were (and, of course, still are) being explored and made available to mass audiences. Ever since Jean Jacques Rousseau called attention to the needs of children and made adults aware that childhood and the process of growing up was worth their involvement, the number of theories concerning childhood learning and development and how to care for and nurture children has multiplied. This century, sometimes called the century of childhood, has seen children become the shuttlecock of whatever theory of child rearing was in fashionable sway, from the regular feeds, no cuddling, firm handling of Truby King and behaviourist J. B. Watson to the 'understand your child' permissive approach of Spock. Each of these theories was very well-meaning and full of good intentions but probably claimed quite a large number of victims – the so called 'Spock marked' child, for instance, self-indulgent and self-centred, ruling the family with his need for self-fulfilment and happiness ever after. But whatever theory happened to be in vogue it became recognised that the child indeed had enormous potential for learning and, in order to realise it, required a great deal more attention from his parents and his environment than had ever been given in the past. Only exceptional parents could provide this for a large family. The small family was seen to be the one with the most advantages where children could get the individual attention that would enable them to benefit from education offered by society.

This century has seen fluctuations in family size from the small family in the 1930s to the slightly larger families of the post-war period, particularly in the States, when many middle-class women opted to have four children rather than two. This was probably the result of post-war advertising to get women back into the home and become consumers (washing machines, washing-up machines, refrigerators, etc.). Another theory propounded to explain the post-war boom, particularly among middle-class American women, was that it was in response to guilty feelings at having so much time on their hands. Their labour-saving devices did so much of the work that used to occupy women in the house (Hoffman & Wyatt 1960). By 1978 mean family size had fallen to 1.8 children per family, from 2.4 children in 1972. Nevertheless, it is doubtful despite these fluctuations whether a return to the large Victorian family of six children (which was then the mean family size) will be seen again in Western nations.

The means of achieving this small family size is the regular use of contraception. Other factors, such as late marriage, delaying the birth of the first child and a fairly high proportion of unmarried, that have been used in some societies, e.g. in Ireland, to control fertility are not in evidence today in Britain. Indeed the reverse is true; more people are marrying younger and having their first babies earlier than ever before. However, child bearing is completed in a short space of time. This obtains for the majority of families in Britain.

THE BENEFITS OF FAMILY PLANNING

Perhaps the chief benefit of family planning is that couples now do have control over their fertility and now have a real choice, not only on family size and family spacing but also on whether to have children at all. Many unintended pregnancies can be avoided if contraception is used consistently. The benefit fo. women has been profound. Women could never hope to enjoy equality with men while they were subjected to the possibility of repeated pregnancies.

Health

Contraception, despite side effects associated with it, has improved the health of both women and children. Having many children and short intervals between births are both directly associated with poor health in mothers and children. Infant mortality rates are higher among children born to women who have large families regardless as to age or social class (Heady & Morris 1959, Butler & Bonham 1963). When births are one year apart the death rate for the child is higher than when the interval is two years. Young mothers under eighteen years show a higher rate of premature births and toxaemia. Pregnancy can mean a high risk to health in a woman suffering from heart and kidney diseases or diabetes.

The example of Aberdeen shows what can be done to improve maternal and child health by promoting contraceptive use through an intensive health education programme. Between 1960 and 1971 there was a drop in the infant mortality rate from 19.2 to 14.5 per 1,000 births, compared with 26.4 for the whole of Scotland in 1960 and 19.6 in 1970. In 1971 there was a further drop to 12.3 per 1000 in Aberdeen, giving one of the lowest rates in the world. The underlying reason for this was the reduction in Aberdeen's high-risk pregnancies (pregnancies in women over thirty-five and those with four or more children) and this in turn was due to the active family planning programme.

Social and emotional

Family planning can improve the marital relationship. In the past, fear of pregnancy often produced sexual difficulties which, in turn, caused marital problems. Effective contraception allows a couple to exercise control over their lives and future; children can be spaced so as not only to prevent fatigue and physical illness in the mother but also to enable the mother to devote more time and care to each individual child. Perseverance with contraception in the sexually active teenager can allow time for emotional maturity to develop.

Economic

Unwanted pregnancy can intensify family poverty, and although poverty itself must be tackled socially and politically, family planning can help the individual family.

Community benefits

Political and Economic Planning (PEP) carried out a study on the costs and benefits of family planning 1972 (Laing 1972). A comparison was made between the supportive costs and the savings that could have been made if contraception had been used to prevent the birth of the 'unwanted' and illegitimate children. It assumed that most illegitimate children are unwanted (which may be questionable). However, what is not questionable is the heavy use of welfare services − 28 per cent of children admitted to long-term (more than six months) care were illegitimate.

PEP also used Cartwright's findings (1970) that the proportion of unwanted births in large families increased from 5 per cent for the second child to 25 per cent for the fourth and 52 per cent for the sixth. Thus the younger children in large families are a major proportion of all unwanted children. PEP found that the fathers of five or more children had more days off work through sickness than the fathers of fewer than five. However, this probably reflects the higher-than-average sickness rates in lower social classes, who also tend to have large families.

PEP concluded that the use of family planning could produce savings for the community. The study ended with the following paragraph: 'It seems particularly desirable that local authorities should consider the total benefits of investment in family planning. At present, the costs of family planning are generally laid on health committees' budgets, whilst other committees' budgets benefit from its provision.'

Avoidance of unintended pregnancies

All the fertility studies done in Britain and America have shown a high incidence of unintended pregnancies which may result in unwanted or regretted children, particularly after the fourth child. While some of the pregnancies were due to method failure and irregular use of contraception, many were due to the failure to use contraception at all. Under half (46 per cent) of the pregnancies in Bone's (1973) study and just over half (52 per cent) in that of Cartwright (1976) were planned in the sense that couples either stopped using birth control to have a child, or definitely intended to get pregnant; 64 per cent of third and 72 per cent of fourth children were unplanned (Bone 1973). A third of all third children and 50 per cent of all fourth children were regretted among mothers studied in 1973 (Cartwright 1976). Those with 1—2 children are more likely to have planned their children than those with 3—4 children (Woolf 1972). By 1975 with improved family planning facilities and increasing availability of abortion the number of regretted pregnancies decreased (Bone 1978, Cartwright 1978). However, it remains evident that there are still groups who are at higher risk than others of having an unwanted pregnancy. These include the wives of manual workers and classes IV and V, those who conceived before marriage and those who conceived or married before the age of twenty (Bone 1978, Cartwright 1978). While it is accepted that unintended and unplanned pregnancies are not synonymous with unwanted children (and vice versa), yet it is not unreasonable to suppose that some of these unintended pregnancies do become unwanted children. They also indicate that though as a society we are moving towards the ideal of contraception being regularly used as a normal and accepted part of sexual relationships, we have not yet reached it. This is clearly attested by the fact that there are more than 100,000 abortions in Britain each year. Studies on women seeking abortion show that a large proportion either do not use contraception or have not used it on the occasion when they became pregnant. Social workers are often involved with the families who are most at risk from unwanted pregnancy and who are less healthy and more socially disadvantaged. Although family planning of itself cannot solve all social problems, nevertheless, it can contribute in a positive way to personal happiness and health. By understanding why some families have particular difficulties with contraception the social worker can offer constructive help to overcome them.

THE SOCIOLOGY AND PSYCHOLOGY
OF CONTRACEPTION AND FAMILY PLANNING

The factors that determine the use or non-use of contraception are similar to those that determine family size and indeed are interchangeable.

1 Those concerned with patterns of living: socio-economic, religion, level of education, cultural.

These also include the attitudes of society (or that particular group to which an individual belongs) towards the idea of family planning and the 'right' family size, what is considered appropriate and what individuals believe is considered appropriate. This can perhaps be summed up as the influence of friends and neighbours and what is considered the 'norm'.

2 Those concerned with contraception itself:

a) acceptance/non-acceptance of the idea of planned parenthood;

b) knowledge of and availability of methods (including costs);

c) attitudes towards the methods themselves;

d) attitudes towards the services providing contraception.

3 Those concerned with the sexual/marital relationship:

a) its stability — the more stable the relationship and the greater the commitment to it, the more likely it is that contraception will be used;

b) expectations of the relationship and attitudes towards male/female and husband/wife roles of each partner. Included here is the 'balance' of the relationship, i.e. who is dominant and who makes the decisions, and also the quality of the relationship, how much care and understanding there is between the partners;

c) attitudes towards sex and acceptance of it for mutual pleasure, rather than solely for procreation. Included here is the way in which each individual takes responsibility for his/her own sexual behaviour;

d) attitudes towards children and how far they are considered to be individual people with their own needs and wishes.

4 Psychological and emotional factors, needs and desires affecting the individual. Pertinent here are feelings concerned with femininity and masculinity and how far these are bound up with the ability to procreate. Anxieties about this prohibit the sustained use of contraception.

Although these factors have been listed separately for the

sake of clarity, in practice they are interrelated; for example, religion affects attitudes to sex, use of contraception and family size. Awareness of these factors and assessment of their relative importance are essential when counselling individuals or couples on contraception.

In an effort to predict future fertility, sociologists have tended to focus on the more tangible factors — social, economic and religious — that influence the use of contraception and choice of family size. Fewer studies have devoted themselves to the more personal (and more difficult to evaluate) influences on fertility control. Rainwater's studies (1960, 1965) are perhaps the best-known of these. They were the first to examine in depth the effects on family size and contraceptive usage of the marital relationship and attitudes towards sex and children. The findings will be looked at in more detail later.

WHY DO PEOPLE HAVE CHILDREN?

Before examining the factors influencing contraceptive usage and family size, remembering it takes two to make a baby and only one to prevent it, the reason why people have children at all needs to be examined. At first sight it may seem impertinent to do so. It is almost automatically assumed that couples will marry and have children. The childless couple in all societies has a negative image. It is often inferred that such couples are either selfish, neurotic or in poor health. Parenthood is considered the norm and the large family is often believed to be less selfish and more caring than the smaller family. These attitudes may be changing nowadays in view of the publicity surrounding over-population (Cartwright 1976). Interestingly, one of the earliest American fertility studies, the Indianapolis study done in the 1940s (Whelpton & Kiser 1958), showed that 6 per cent of females and 8 per cent of males recalled having wanted no children.

In the past, when life was short, infant mortality rates were high and hands were needed in the fields, great emphasis was placed on fertility and procreation. Having children was considered a duty both to the family (to carry on the family name and inherit property) and to society, regardless of the individual's feelings. To be fruitful and multiply, the injunction of all religions, was essential for the survival of the species. Barrenness (or inability to have children, a condition usually blamed on the woman) was considered a curse and grounds for ending a marriage. These attitudes are still prevalent in underdeveloped countries. In Africa, for example, a marriage is not considered complete without children. Furthermore, for many African tribes children ensure some degree of immortality since they are considered to incorporate some of the attributes of the recently dead (the so-called 'living dead'). Thus having children becomes a sacred duty (Mbiti 1969). It is extremely unusual to find an African (even one who is a Christian) requesting sterilisation or agreeing to it even if it is strongly advised on medical grounds.

Religious influence is still an important factor for those who are strict observers. For example, both British and American fertility studies have found that Catholics tend to want and to have more children than Protestants. Thus couples may have children to conform to the expectations of society and of their religion. However, now that there is a real choice about whether or not to have children (less societal and religious pressure, effective contraception) the reasons for having children probably have more to do with individual psychology and family dynamics. Elucidating what are the most significant factors for individual couples can be difficult – for example, do women have an innate need to have children? Pohlman (1969) concluded that 'very little is known for sure about possible innate needs to be a mother. If such needs exist they have been heavily overlaid by cultural learning. Their very existence is difficult to isolate and demonstrate.' Freudian analytical theory has suggested a number of possible reasons, often unconscious, for wanting children: a need to prove virility or fertility, competition with a parent of the same sex, a son as a penis substitute or as a substitute lover. The first baby may be the result of a hostile desire to replace the mother. The first child is also evidence of adultness and independence from parents. Having a larger or smaller family may be an attempt to outdo mother or siblings or spouse's siblings. There may be a wish to recreate one's own actual family of origin or to create the family one would like to have belonged to. Parents may exert pressure on their own children to produce grandchildren. Children can be seen as a punishment for sex. Having children can be a form of self love, or an extension of the ego, narcissism invested in the child. This seems to occur particularly in those individuals who have grown up deprived of love and with low self-esteem. It is also seen characteristically in some teenage girls, particularly those who have been in care and some mothers of large families. In these situations the children may be used to 'mother the mother' or placed in the husband role where there are unsatisfactory adult relationships. Couples may have children to cement a relationship or marriage, or to prevent a marriage from breaking up. Life can be lived vicariously through children. Children can be used to fulfil the failed ambitions of the parents. Parents can project dependency needs on to the child: by taking care of the child the parent really takes care of him/herself. Children are proof of virility and feminity, maleness and femaleness. Children may be seen as a means of preventing ageing ('children keep you young') and keeping the idea of death at bay. Individuals, uncertain of their role and identity, may have a child for this very reason, that is, to define themselves and to have someone who needs and is dependent on them. Being a mother, particularly in lower socio-economic groups, can be the reason for living. Children, by providing action and stimulation, can be a relief from boredom and loneliness. They are an investment in and for the future. Rearing children can be seen as a creative occupation.

The actual number of children a couple or individual have is determined by the factors mentioned above, but there are others, as well. Many couples who have a boy and a girl are content to stop at two, whereas, if the children are of the same sex they may want to go on until they have a child of the opposite sex. This can take on an almost pathological aspect with couples having very large families in an effort to obtain the son or daughter. If they are successful the only son or only daughter often has to pay a heavy price in the form of stereo-typed role-playing for that sex. The little girl may be expected to show exaggerated femininity and the boy exaggerated masculinity, and characteristics of the other sex are often sternly repressed.

Some women only feel needed if they have a baby in their arms. As soon as the baby becomes a toddler they have another baby to replace it. They can cope with the relatively uncomplic-ated demands of a baby, who may be seen as an extension of themselves (part of self-love and self-care) but as soon as the baby becomes a toddler expressing his individuality and independence, the mother feels empty and bereft.

Certain collusive relationships within marriage can determine family size. For example, a large family may increase the de-pendence of the wife on the husband, a situation they may both wish for. Marriages where there is little sharing of activities or decision-making, where the roles of husband and wife are segregated, often result in large families (Rainwater 1960, Cartwright 1976).

Women who equate femininity with fertility and have stereo-typically feminine concepts tend to have significantly larger families than those with relatively masculine self-concepts (Clarkson 1970). Success in planning a family has been found to depend on the 'presence of an emotionally stable, self confident well satisfied personality' (Whelpton & Kiser 1958).

The number of children born outside marriage has been increasing steadily in all Western nations since the 1950s. (There has been a slight fall in recent years in Britain, owing to the liberalisation of the abortion law.) These births are excluded from fertility studies, possibly because although the numbers are increasing they still form a small proportion of all births. Ten per cent of births in Britain are illegitimate. (The ratio in inner city areas is much higher (1 in 5 or 6.) The causality of illegitimacy is complex — a mixture of social, cultural and individual factors. It cannot be divorced from the issues surrounding young people and sex. This and illegitimacy will be examined in Chapter 13. Whatever moral viewpoint is taken of illegitimacy (and none is implied here) the one-parent family, especially where the parent is young, is a particularly disadvantaged one in society.

To sum up, the reasons for parenthood are many and varied and not necessarily the result of an informed and thoughtful decision nor even for perhaps the best reason of actually liking children. In ante-natal clinics where every care is given to physical wellbeing, it is perhaps surprising that almost no attention is paid to mental wellbeing and exploration of attitudes towards children. It could be argued that such an exploration might help those potential and actual parents who have unrealistic and idealised expectations of their children which in turn may lead to child abuse (physical and emotional) when these expectations are not realised. Sex education in schools should encompass preparation for parenthood.

WHAT SIZE FAMILY DO PEOPLE WANT?

Both British (Woolf 1967, 1972; Cartwright 1970, 1976, 1978) and American (Freedman *et al.* 1959; Whelpton *et al.* 1966; Westoff *et al.* 1961, 1963; Westoff & Bumpass 1970; Ryder &

Westoff 1971) fertility studies show that the majority of married couples, regardless of social class or religion, *want* 2—4 children. There has been a definite decline in the number of children thought ideal (i.e. if there are no financial worries). Most couples want their children in the first ten years of marriage.

Most couples do have ideas about family size at marriage, but these are not fixed and are often modified in the light of experience with children. Thus family desires are best examined after the birth of the second child or five years of marriage (Westoff & Bumpass 1970, Woolf 1972); 'fertility affects fertility'. The number of couples having three or more children, regardless of socio-economic group, is falling. In all the studies done so far the largest families are found among the semi-skilled and unskilled. Women in this group are more likely to be pregnant at marriage, to have a pregnancy as a teenager and to marry younger. They also have more unintended pregnancies. Women who come from large families tend to leave school early, marry young and have large families. Catholics tend to want and have larger families than Protestants. However, a British study (Peel & Carr 1976) on a nationally representative sample of women (1,678) married in the winter of 1970-71 showed that although more Roman Catholic wives than others thought 3—4 children ideal, 54 per cent affirmed that 2 was the best number.

The desirability of contraception has gained greater acceptance, though some couples do not use it after marriage and only use it consistently and regularly after the desired family size has been reached. The use of contraception is affected by education — the poorly educated tend to delay using contraception until they have three or more children and they tend to use it less regularly. Thus the avoidance of unintended pregnancies is not just a matter of cheap, effective and convenient methods of birth control but is a *'matter of establishing the habitual use of contraception as a normal and accepted part of married life'* (Whelpton *et al.* 1966).

9
Fertility and Poverty

Before discussing the relationship between fertility and poverty it should be noted that not all poor families in Britain are large ones. Of the 460,000 families receiving Supplementary Benefit only 60,000 had four or more children (Hansard 30 March 1979, Written Answers). However, large families are likely to be poor. Rearing children is a costly business and the more children there are the less money there is likely to be available for each child, despite allowances and benefits. Further, children in a large family are disadvantaged from the point of view of physical growth and as regards educational achievement, whatever their position in the birth order (Davie *et al.* 1972).

As we have seen, most married couples (and this includes most poor families) do not want large families. Yet more poor families end up by having more children than they expected or wanted than other socio-economic groups. Why is this? The short, simple answer is that the poor tend to delay using contraception until they already have three or more children and when they do use contraception they use it less effectively. It is important to understand why this should be, since 'the choice couples make in their efforts to control conception has a fatefulness for their lives together that few other choices in marriage have' (Rainwater 1965). Cost and availability of contraceptives must obviously have played a role in the past, though this is perhaps less of a deterrent since free contraception became available from clinics in 1974 and from GPs in 1975. Are there other factors responsible? The poor are often seen by society as acting 'irrationally' by having large families that they cannot afford. They are also seen as living in the present with no thought for the future. Certainly more women (25 per cent) from social classes IV and V did not know how many children they wanted compared to other social classes (17 per cent: Cartwright 1976). Various attempts have been made to explain lower working-class (i.e. semi-skilled and unskilled) behaviour. Askham (1975) has fully reviewed current theories regarding such behaviour. Briefly, some authors (Cohen & Hodges 1963, Lewis 1966) see working-class behaviour as part of a separate culture — the 'culture of poverty' — which has values and norms different from the rest of society. At society level there is little integration and participation. At the family level there is a trend towards female-centred families in conjunction with authoritarianism. At the individual level there are feelings of helplessness, dependence, inferiority, and an inability to plan for the future. This includes family planning. Other authors (Titmuss 1962, Rosenthal 1968) stress the situation the poor find themselves in — the material deprivation and lack of educational opportunity. The inability to plan ahead is seen more in terms of the 'low estimates of opportunities and high expectations of risk which the poor have rather than a supposed inability to defer gratification' (Miller & Riesman 1961). Askham herself favours an 'adaptational' explanation. For couples who feel they have no control over their future, planning ahead including planning a family may appear either irrelevant or impossible. Consequently they do not plan and a large family may be the result.

Support was found in Askham's study for two patterns of behaviour to explain why the lower working class are less efficient users of birth control:

a) there is a lack of concern for the consequences of achieving a large family;

b) the attitudes to material wellbeing and status are such that the effect of a large family on their standard of living would not be taken seriously into consideration. However, not one of the 91 families studied had more than six children. Furthermore, there are few families with five or more children in Aberdeen. The reason for this is the active family planning programme initiated by Sir Dugald Baird (former Professor of Obstetrics and Gynaecology in Aberdeen) and the local MoH, Dr MacGregor. They were ahead of the rest of Britain in setting up free family-planning facilities, combined with an extensive programme of education carried out by health visitors. Sir Dugald Baird used a more liberal interpretation of the existing law with regard to abortion and he performed sterilisation on those women who requested it and offered it routinely to all women with four or more children. The fact that there are so few families with five or more children shows that the poor can indeed 'adapt' and have smaller families, provided good family-planning facilities are available.

Two key American studies on fertility and the poor (Rainwater 1960, 1965) noted the relevance to the use of contraception of feelings of apathy and lack of control. In addition these studies explored the effect on the use of contraception of sexual and marital relationships together with attitudes towards children. The findings are discussed in some detail here since in the author's experience they are relevant to some of the families referred to the domiciliary family planning service. These families also tend to be involved with the social services.

The subjects had intensive interviews covering socio-economic status, background of wives and their husbands (occupation, education, housing, etc.), family relations and attitudes towards children, role of motherhood and fatherhood, attitudes towards pregnancy, methods of birth control, sexual relations before and after marriage, awareness of their own and spouse's sexual desires and the importance of these and the satisfactions and dissatisfactions with sexual relations. They were also asked about their attitudes towards helping agencies and professional people in instructing couples about contraceptives.

On the basis of his findings Rainwater was able to divide his sample into effective and ineffective users of contraception. The ineffective users he was able to subdivide into a 'do nothing' group, sporadic users, and the late desperate planners. The effective users (largely skilled manual) did not necessarily plan from the beginning (they usually had 1—2 children before using contraception), but once they did start they managed to use contraception effectively. The effective users tended to be closer to middle-class patterns in insisting on the virtues of 'niceness', 'cleanliness' and 'financial stability' (Rainwater's terms). They also had stronger perceptions of children as individuals. There was rational discussion about contraception between husband and wife. Sex tended to be enjoyed by both parties (pattern of mutuality). The ineffective users (largely semi-skilled & unskilled manual), on the other hand, found life unpredictable. Fate and God's will tended to be blamed for the repeated pregnancies. Thus everything depended on 'luck'. The ineffective women users had a greater sense of estrangement and isolation from their husbands, whom they found impulsive and given to inexplicable anger. The ineffective men users found women 'emotional', demanding, irrational and always wanting affection. Sex was regarded as a 'getting on and off' experience. The sexual attitudes of ineffective women users were either ones of active rejection in which the woman reacted to sex with fear, disgust and anxiety or passive rejection (the 'repressive compromisers') who denied any sexual feelings. A frequent comment from such women was 'sex is no trouble to me'. By denying any sexual feelings they hoped their husbands would moderate their desires. The woman's rejection of sexuality often carried with it a rejection of responsibility for contraception; 'he gets the pleasure, he should do something'. Thus the women failed to separate their negative feelings about intercourse from their own self-interest in not having more children, since many had children they did not want. Among the ineffective users children tended to be seen as pleasurable objects valued for the day-to-day sense of wellbeing they provided rather than as individuals.

Among Rainwater's 'do nothing' group were some Roman Catholics whose ambivalence towards contraception did not prevent them experimenting with methods but did prevent sustained use. For the sporadic users the methods of birth control (this was before the pill and IUD) were too much trouble. The 'do nothing' group and the sporadic users tended to become the late desperate planners; that is, a breaking-point was reached (the woman's health or the family budget) and the woman requested sterilisation or made the man use sheaths regularly. The men and women found the idea of being visited at home by family planning personnel acceptable, a point of particular relevance to domiciliary family planning services.

The second study (Rainwater 1965) explored, among other things, the conjugal role relationship and its effect on the use of contraception. Use was made of Bott's concepts of conjugal relationships. Bott (1957) described conjugal role relationships as ranging along a continuum from the jointly organised (shared activity, task can be done by either husband or wife) to the highly segregated (husband and wife take different activities and tasks and conform to a more stereotyped role of man and woman). Rainwater found a preponderance of segregated role relationships among the unskilled working class. This was associated with ineffective use of contraception and negative attitudes to sex on the part of the woman. Contraception was not discussed. The jointly organised couples were found more among the skilled manual class. They tended to discuss contraception and were more effective users.

Other studies have confirmed Rainwater's findings and shown that where household tasks are shared there is a tendency for couples to have smaller families (less than four children) and for the last pregnancy to have been intended (Cartwright 1976, Woolf 1972). This was because there was greater discussion about birth control, sex and the number of children wanted. Among the working class the proportion of women who had not discussed such matters was from 7 per cent of those with one child to 55 per cent of those with five or more children (Cartwright 1976).

Regardless of what theory is held to be the most appropriate to explain lower working-class behaviour, the effect of poor fertility control is to make their situation worse and to increase feelings of despair, hopelessness and apathy. Professionals working with such families need to guard against pessimism. This may hinder them from trying to help such families exercise control over their fertility. Finally, evidence that poor families can and do respond to economic changes is seen in the Registrar General's figures for 1970-72. While the overall number of births fell by 8 per cent the decline in social classes IV and V was 16 per cent; that is twice as great as for the population as a whole!

10
Birth Control Services Available on the National Health Service

The history of the modern birth control movement begins after the publication of Malthus' famous essay on population in 1790 which put forward the idea that population was increasing more rapidly than food supplies since population increases geometrically and food supply increases arithmetically. Malthus recommended late marriages and abstinence as a solution. During the early nineteenth century thousands of handbills were circulated on contraception. By the late nineteenth century there was a retail trade in contraceptives including rubber letters (condoms), the diaphragm or cap, and vaginal pessaries. Abortion was widely resorted to, although accurate figures cannot be given (Potts *et al.* 1977).

In 1921 Marie Stopes, a geologist, opened the first birth control clinic in Britain (in London). A growing concern with infant and maternal mortality allied with feminism led to the setting up of welfare clinics and encouraged the birth control movement. Between 1921 and 1930, five separate birth control societies were formed to open clinics. 'Children by choice not chance' was their slogan. In 1930 these societies merged to become the National Birth Control Council. There were then just twenty birth control clinics. The method recommended by the clinics was the cap.

In 1939 the National Birth Control Council became the Family Planning Association, which concerned itself with the whole problem of fertility including sub-fertility. By now there were sixty-nine clinics. In 1943 the first centre for the investigation of male sub-fertility was started in London, as was the first psychosexual clinic, called the Marital Difficulties Clinic. Formal training in contraceptive techniques for doctors and nurses was established to take place in designated clinics. No training was done in medical schools at that time.

In 1955 the FPA received official recognition when the then Minister of Health, Iain Macleod, made an official visit. By 1958 the number of clinics had increased to 292.

In 1959 work began on domiciliary services. The pill was approved for use in the clinics in 1961, the coil in 1965. In 1967 the National Health Service Family Planning Act gave local health authorities permissive powers to give birth control advice without regard to marital status, to social as well as medical cases, using voluntary organisations such as the FPA as their agent. It was at this time that the National Council of the FPA empowered clinics to give advice to the unmarried. In 1964 Helen Brook had set up the Brook Clinics in London, Bristol and Birmingham, specifically to give advice to the unmarried. These clinics are still functioning. The Marie Stopes Clinic continues to function in Whitfield Street, London, under new management as the Marie Stopes Centre, providing a comprehensive birth control service, including vasectomy.

From April 1974 family planning became part of the National Health Service and advice and supplies were free from the clinics for married and single alike. The domiciliary services, of which there were about 140, were taken over in April 1975. The clinics were handed over to the Area Health Authorities in October 1976. In 1975 GPs began to offer family planning services under the National Health Service.

The man or woman, regardless of age or marital status, who wants advice about contraception can go to a clinic or to a general practitioner.

Clinics are usually held in child welfare clinics, and are of two main types: one for the pill, cap and sheath, the other for IUD fitting as this needs special equipment. There are also special young people's clinics giving birth control advice and counselling to young people. Included here are the Brook Clinics for young people. (For addresses, see p. 324.) The needs of the young will be considered later. Appointments at clinics may have to be made in advance. There is also an increasing number of hospital family planning clinics, held in the maternity department. Local facilities may vary; clinic times and location can be obtained from the Area or District Health Authority. Contraceptives (the pill, cap, sheath) are available directly from the clinic. Pregnancy testing is available at many clinics which also usually offer counselling for unwanted pregnancy. Counselling is also available for male and female sterilisation and referral can be made to the appropriate clinic or hospital department.

General practitioners can be seen in surgery times. Some GPs offer a comprehensive birthcontrol service apart from prescription of the sheath. Others offer a more limited service prescribing the pill and referring their patients to family planning clinics for the coil or cap. Women seeing a GP get the pills he prescribes from a chemist.

The choice of the source of advice is entirely up to the individual or couple concerned and they may change their source of advice if they so wish from GP to clinic or vice versa. Advice and supplies are free from either source.

The Domiciliary Family Planning Service is a specialised service which visits women at home for contraceptive advice after referral by a health visitor or social worker (see chapter 12).

PROCEDURE AT A CLINIC

A case card is usually filled out by a lay worker with the woman's name, address and details about the GP. She is then seen by the nurse who discusses the method of birth control and takes a medical, menstrual and obstetric history, then weighs her and takes her blood pressure and gives her leaflets to read. The doctor sees her next, reviews her medical history and discusses the methods further.

If the woman selects the pill (provided there are no medical contra-indications) her breasts and vagina are examined and a cervical smear test is done. This is painless and takes only a few minutes. The woman returns to the nurse for teaching and to get her supply of pills. She is seen after six weeks; then, if all is well, every three months for the first year and every six months thereafter.

If the cap is chosen, the doctor does a routine vaginal examination and fits the cap. The woman is then taught how to use it. Usually she practises at home with a cap, then returns the following week to see if she is comfortable with it and knows exactly how to fit it. If this is satisfactory she is seen again in six months.

If the IUD is chosen, the woman is referred to an IUD clinic. The woman is shown the coil to be fitted and taught how to check that it is in place. It is usually fitted either during or at the end of a period for ease of fitting and also because it is less likely that the woman will be pregnant. It takes only a few minutes to fit a coil. The failure rate is discussed and the woman instructed what to do if she misses a period or has very heavy periods or is unable to feel the threads in the vagina. The woman is seen again after six weeks to check the coil and, if all is well, is seen again in six months and then yearly.

Sheaths can be obtained free of charge at family planning clinics without seeing the doctor.

If sterilisation is requested, a medical, obstetric and menstrual history is taken, with a medical history for the men. The nature and finality of the operation is explained. Counselling is given to ascertain that the sterilisation operation is not being used as a solution to other problems and that one partner is not putting pressure on the other to have it done.

ATTITUDES TO THE FP SERVICES

In 1976 2.36 million women in England and Wales were registered with their GPs for family planning and 1.54 million women attended the 1837 family planning clinics in England and Wales (Hansard 9 December 1977).

Studies done on family planning services during the late sixties and early seventies (Cartwright 1970, Bone 1973) showed that middle-class women tended to go to the clinics for advice while working-class women used the GP. Criticisms were made of both services — clinics were too few, too busy and in-accessible, while GPs often only offered one method — the pill — without adequate explanations and frequently no examin-ation (a significant factor, since this may influence perseverance with the pill because of anxieties surrounding it). A later study (Bone 1978) showed more women of all social classes going to the GP rather than the clinic for advice — 23 per cent as com-pared to 17 per cent. Nevertheless, it appears that the gap is narrowing between social classes in their use of both services, particularly among those married recently. Thus among couples married between 1971 and 1975, 26 per cent of social classes I and II used the GP and 24 per cent the clinic, compared to 25 per cent of social classes IV and V using the GP and 22 per cent the clinic. It used to be thought that middle-class women, being more literate, articulate and mobile, were more likely to use the clinics since they felt they would get more specialised help and were not ashamed to be seen there. For working-class women, on the other hand, the GP was seen as more con-venient and less embarrassing (since no one need know why you were there), and there was less likelihood of a vaginal examination which many working-class women feared (and continue to fear). It may be that the increasing acceptability of contraception both privately and publicly is allowing all women greater freedom of choice of FP services. Certainly clinics are known to the writer whose clientele is exclusively working-class and to which women themselves are extremely loyal. So much depends on the welcome, attention and care which the woman both expects to receive and, in reality, does receive.

11
Methods of Birth Control

Nowadays, a woman's fertility extends from 12 years (the average age of the menarche (in the nineteenth century the average age was 17 years) to 50 years (the average age of the menopause). A woman's fertility is said to reach a peak around 23 years and thereafter to decline slowly. A man's fertility extends from about 14 years till well into old age. The fertility of any one couple can only be known for certain retrospectively, that is after they have become pregnant and with regard to the time it has taken to become pregnant. This is one of the difficult issues that have to be faced by couples. Thus some couples adopt a 'wait and see' policy and either do not use contraceptives at all or use them haphazardly. This 'wait and see', although found in all social classes and cultures, is particularly noticeable in lower socio-economic groups and in certain cultures such as Asian, West Indian and African. Yet other couples will use contraception conscientiously prior to the first pregnancy and then find difficulty in conceiving (this refers to couples where this difficulty is unrelated to the method used). About 10 per cent of all couples are infertile. Fertility, of course, can be affected subsequently by pelvic infections (secondary infertility). Thus couples lie on a 'fertility spectrum' that ranges from the very fertile (a baby every year) to the completely infertile.

The birth control methods to be described are the orthodox ones together with their advantages and disadvantages. There are, of course, unorthodox ones said by folklore to be efficacious, such as hoping for the best, 'it can't happen to me', having sex standing up, urinating after intercourse, jumping up and down, sneezing, coughing, all of which seem to rely on getting rid of the sperm. Unfortunately for these methods, the sperm takes only 90 seconds to get into the uterus (it has to be quick in order to survive the lethal acid vaginal secretions). Other 'methods' are drinking cold water, to flush out the sperms, and not climaxing at the same time as the men (a belief prevalent among West Indian women).

Despite scare stories about methods, particularly the pill and coil, Tietze (1977) found that up to the age of thirty the risk to life among those *not* using contraception from pregnancy and childbirth is far in excess of that experienced by users of *any* method. Vessey (1978) gave a figure of 2—4 deaths per 100,000 per year for each method of birth control together with any accidental pregnancies for the age group 20—34 years. For the age group 35—44 years the mortality risk experienced by pill users was 20 deaths per 100,000; for coil or cap users 2 per 100,000.

The health of the woman is least affected at all ages by relying on the sheath or diaphragm backed up by abortion.

Couples may use two methods in conjunction, e.g. sheaths and chemicals, withdrawal and chemicals; or may use a variety of methods, eventually settling on one; or may pursue the same method throughout sexual life where this method has proved reliable and acceptable.

Effectiveness of any method is usually measured in pregnancies per hundred women years. This refers to the number of pregnancies occurring in a hundred women using the method for one year. However, effectiveness depends on regular use and this in turn depends on the motivation and acceptance of the method.

Coitus Interruptus

Variously described as withdrawal, being careful, discharging (by West Indians), pulling out, getting off at Crewe if you are on the way to Glasgow. Curiously, it is often not considered as a method of birth control by the couples who use it. Thus a specific question has to be asked, 'Is your husband being careful?' It was probably the most commonly used birth control method and is probably still used at one time or another by most couples and especially by young people first starting intercourse. Cartwright (1970) found that 45 per cent of couples had used it at some time.

What is it? The man withdraws his penis from the vagina before ejaculation so that the ejaculate with its sperms is released outside the vagina.

Advantages It is free, easy to use, and does not require medical advice. Women are often proud when their husbands or partners use this method. 'He takes care of me' is a frequent comment made.

Disadvantages The man has to exercise much self-control to be aware when the ejaculation process starts to occur. The woman may find it hard to relax and enjoy intercourse because of anxiety about whether her partner will successfully withdraw. As one woman succinctly put it, 'I says — don't let yourself go or you'll forget to keep an eye on him.' Thus it does impose a constraint on the sexual act at its most pleasurable moment and may cause sexual frustration in both partners. However, many couples seem to cope successfully with it and it is only when a pregnancy has resulted from using this method that the couple may become tense if they go on using it.

Effectiveness This is difficult to estimate but in one American study the failure rate was 10 pregnancies per 100 women years.

The sheath

It is variously known as the condom (from an apocryphal story that it was named after a certain Colonel Condom at the court of Charles II), the French letter (in France, *capot anglais*), as Johnnies, rubbers, or protectives, or by its brand name 'Durex' (though if this is requested in Australia, sellotape will be given). It remains the second most used male method. One company manufactures 150,000,000 per year. It is mentioned in Pepys's *Diary*. In the 1870s sheaths became widely available and were made of rubber. Today they are made of fine latex 0.065–0.075 mm. thick. They are made in assorted colours and attempts are being made to package them more attractively. Sheaths which are lubricated with spermicide are now available.

It is a tube that covers the entire length of the penis and is teat-ended or round-ended. It should be used once only and care should be taken to remove the sheath when intercourse is finished so that it does not slip off into the vagina as this may result in pregnancy. It has no other effect and cannot get lost.

Advantages It is easy to use and does not need medical advice. It lessens the transmission of venereal disease, provided it is used from the beginning of sexual contact. Bold and humorous advertising in Sweden has been correlated with an increasing sale of condoms and a decline in venereal disease. Clinical experience shows that men who use the sheath conscientiously are often more concerned with their partner's welfare than those who do not.

Disadvantages It is expensive. Some couples find it aesthetically unacceptable. Sex may not be as enjoyable. Some men are allergic to rubber and they may develop a rash on the penis and scrotum; there are special sheaths for such men. Sheaths may burst with rough handling. Occasionally men with anxiety about their fertility or a need to punish or control the woman may deliberately sabotage the sheath (by putting a hole in it) to get the woman pregnant. Thus from the woman's point of view the sheath may be unsatisfactory as it is not under her control.

Effectiveness 2—4 pregnancies per 100 women years.

Cap and cream

Caps are made of rubber and were first devised by a Dutchman called Mensinga in 1885 (hence their other name, Dutch cap).

There are two main types of cap — the vaginal cap or diaphragm which covers the neck of the womb and front wall of the vagina, and the cervical cap which covers only the neck of the womb. The latter used to be prescribed for the woman who had had several children, since she had poor vaginal muscle tone and could not retain the vaginal cap. Both have to be used with spermicidal cream. The woman is taught how to use the cap. It can be inserted about two hours before intercourse and then left for six hours afterwards. This allows time for the sperm to be killed by the cream. The correctly fitted cap should be comfortable; neither the woman nor the man should be aware of it. The cap needs to be checked every six months at the clinic, as it may be misshapen and therefore not fit properly, and the rubber may have perished. After use it is washed in warm water (not detergents), stored in a container and regularly checked for holes.

Advantages It is safe. It does not affect health or have side effects.

Disadvantages It has to be fitted by a doctor. It does need a certain amount of forethought, which some women find puts them off sex. Also some women find their bodies distasteful and do not like inserting fingers into their vaginas. The method needs privacy.

Effectiveness 2—2.5 pregnancies per 100 women years (Kelsey & Wiggins 1974). Thus it is a reliable method of birth control.

Spermicides

These should not be used on their own as their failure rate is quite high. (However, they are used by about 10 per cent of couples as their sole method, and are better than no method at all.) They come in the form of aerosol foams, creams, jellies and pessaries, and need to be inserted in the vagina just before intercourse. They protect for about an hour. They are available from clinics or chemists.

Advantages They are easy to use, and no medical advice is needed.

Disadvantages They are not very effective on their own. They may be messy and cause vaginal irritation.

Effectiveness Tablets are least effective, foams slightly more so. There have been no adequate studies, but figures of 15—37 pregnancies per 100 women years have been quoted.

Safe period, rhythm method

This method is based on the fact that during a certain part of the menstrual cycle a woman is less likely to conceive than at others because ovulation generally occurs only once in the cycle, namely about 12—16 days *before* the next menstrual period and is available for fertilisation by the sperm for about twenty-four hours. The sperm is capable of fertilising the ovum for about forty-eight hours. Although theoretically a period of only about three days in each cycle should be avoided for intercourse, in practice intercourse itself may precipitate the release of an egg. Thus as a rough rule intercourse is *relatively* safe for about three days *after* a period and for about ten days *before* the next period. It is the only method advocated by the Roman Catholic Church. Only about 15 per cent of couples use it as their sole method.

Advantages It does not affect health.

Disadvantages It is unreliable. Intercourse is limited to certain times so that it requires more self-control than other methods.

Effectiveness If intercourse is limited to the time after ovulation (i.e. before the next period is due) the failure rate is 6.6 per 100 women years. If before ovulation, then 19.8 — 40 pregnancies per 100 women years will occur.

The Pill: Oral Contraceptive

The pill, more than any other method, can take the credit for the sexual revolution, since it is practically 100 per cent safe as a contraceptive method if taken correctly, and is not directly concerned with the sexual act itself. People also feel freer to discuss, evaluate and be critical of it. The pill gives women a control over their fertility not previously known. It was obvious given previous attitudes towards sexuality, particularly female sexuality, that this would cause anxiety and concern. The numerous articles in newspapers confirm that we have yet to learn to live with the pill and its implications. It has been known since the 1930s that sex hormones could inhibit the formation of the egg and its release (ovulation). But not until 1950, with the discovery of new steroids, which could be given by mouth without undesirable effects, could they be used. The dosage of hormones used in the late fifties and early sixties was far higher than is necessary to inhibit ovulation. Work is continuing on the pill to lower the dose without altering its effectiveness. It has been available on prescription since 1961 in Britain. About 3 million women of child-bearing age are taking the pill in the UK, that is 1 in 5 women, and about 50 million around the world.

Although hormones can suppress the formation of sperm in men and are therefore effective for contraceptive purposes, the side effects, such as the loss of interest in sex, or nausea with alcohol, prohibit their use.

The combined pill

This is made up of oestrogen and progesterone hormones and is the one most commonly used. It is 100 per cent effective when taken properly. It is taken for 20, 21 or 22 days by mouth. The commonest require 21 days followed by an interval of 7 days when uterine bleeding occurs. There are about thirty different kinds of combined pills with slightly differing hormones and varying amounts in each type, though since the Committee for Safety of Drugs (now the Committee on Safety of Medicines (CSM)) reported on the side effects of the pill in 1968 no pill contains more than 0.05 mg of oestrogen (this being the part of the pill responsible for thrombosis). The newer pills contain 0.03 mg of oestrogen. It is not possible, at present, to select the pill to suit the woman's apparent hormonal make-up, though this has been tried, as most women react in quite individual ways to the pill. However, doctors working at family planning clinics usually have an extensive knowledge of the pill so that when a woman has certain side effects the doctor will know which different pill to prescribe. The combined pill suppresses ovulation by altering the hormone feedback to the master hormone gland (the pituitary gland) which is situated in the base of the brain. In this respect the pill mimics pregnancy, hence certain similar side effects (a woman does not ovulate during pregnancy).

Advantages It is effective, easy to use and does not interfere with the spontaneity of the sex act. Many women experience a sense of wellbeing. Premenstrual tension, painful periods, irregular or prolonged periods are all helped by the pill. Fertility usually returns immediately the pill is stopped, in the majority of women. Periods are lighter and usually begin 2—3 days after the last pill is taken. If the woman becomes pregnant as a result of not taking the pill properly, it does not harm the foetus (Ambani 1977). It is safe to have intercourse at any time in the month including the seven pill-free days.

Disadvantages It needs medical advice and the woman needs to remember to take it regularly. (If one pill is forgotten it can be taken the next morning.) Thirty-six hours are allowed between pills, except with the very low oestrogen (0.03mg) pills.

It has both major and minor side effects. Minor side effects include nausea, weight gain, sore breasts, headaches, absent periods, breakthrough bleeding, depression and vaginal infection. These are usually improved by changing the pill. Loss of interest in sex is sometimes quoted as a side effect though the evidence is not conclusive. Major side effects include a rise in blood pressure and blood clots in the lung, brain and heart. Death may result. Absolute contra-indications to taking the pill include previous thrombosis, cancer, high blood pressure, severe heart and kidney disease and defects in liver function.

Careful supervision is needed for those with asthma, diabetes, epilepsy and a past history of depression or severe migraine and those who smoke, are overweight or have a family history of a close relative dying of heart disease under fifty-five. The pill should be stopped one month before and one month after an operation. It should be used with caution in young girls who have not established regular menstrual cycles and those girls who have anorexia nervosa. There is no evidence so far that the pill causes cancer. The pill has been found to protect against benign breast lumps. Varicose veins are not in themselves a contra-indication to the pill, though women often think they are. Where the varicose veins are severe the woman should be advised to have them treated before going on the pill.

The risk of dying of heart attacks and strokes is thought to be five times greater for women who take the pill than for those who do not. The risk appears to be concentrated in women over thirty-five years, those who have taken the pill for five years or more continuously and those who smoke (RGGP Study 1977, Vessey 1977). However, the Committee on Safety of Medicines (CSM) commented that the numbers in the studies are too small to allow precise conclusions to be reached about the overall risk of using oral contraceptives. Also in view of the fact that during the course of these studies major changes have occurred in the composition of oral contraceptives the Committee did not think it necessary as yet for any change in the warnings and precautions for oral contraceptives. Almost 80 per cent of the women studied were taking pills which contained 0.05 mg oestrogen. Nowadays about 40 per cent of women taking the pill take the smaller (0.03 mg) dose of oestrogen (Vessey 1978).

In women whose periods do not return to normal after stopping the pill there is greater difficulty in getting pregnant. These women can be helped with hormone treatment. It must be remembered that a woman's fertility is unknown if she goes on to the pill before any pregnancies.

The Mini-Pill — single-hormone pill or progesterone only pill

This pill is made up of one hormone — progesterone. It is taken daily without a break. It does not prevent the formation and release of the egg, and is therefore not 100 per cent effective. It alters the nature of the mucus plug in the neck of the womb by keeping it thick so that sperms find it difficult to swim through. The failure rate is 2 per 100 women years (roughly 98 per cent effective). It comes in packs of 28, 35 or 42. It does *not* cause thrombosis because it does not contain oestrogen and hence can be used by women with a history of thrombosis. It can also be taken by women with high blood pressure. It does not interfere with lactation and hence can be used by women who are breast feeding. (The combined pill may inhibit breast feeding, though it does not always do so.) One unfortunate side effect is that the periods may be irregular, either occurring with greater frequency or with prolonged gaps.

Injectables

These are 3 or 6 monthly injections given intramuscularly of a progesterone (trade name Depoprovera). The injection gives 100 per cent protection, though periods may be irregular or absent. The return of fertility may be delayed by a few months after the injections have ceased. It has similar side effects to the combined pill but less risk of thrombosis.

It has not been officially recognised as a long-term contraceptive in this country (though it has been used in the under-developed countries). Its use has been sanctioned for three months in women who have been immunised against German measles and for women whose husbands have just had a vasectomy. Individual doctors can (and do) use it in special cases of women who need contraceptive protection but are dissatisfied with the other methods (Wilson 1976, 1978). Women who use it need careful counselling and follow-up.

Figure 1: The Intra-uterine Device: the Coil

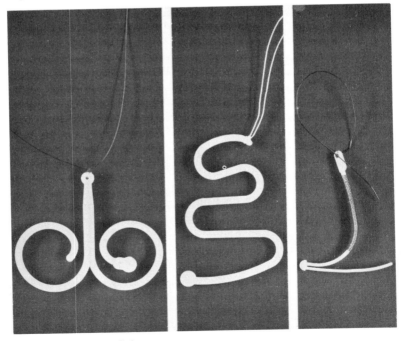

Coils shown at actual size.

There are many different shapes and sizes of intra-uterine devices — see Fig. 1. The reason for this is the search for an effective device with the least side effects. The most commonly used device is the Lippes loop, available since 1962. They are made of polythene impregnated with barium sulphate so that they will show up on X-ray. Polythene has 'memory', that is, it will recoil into its original shape. The newer devices have a copper wire wound round one arm. The metal is the contraceptive. These are the Copper 7 or Gravigard and Copper T.

Mode of action This is not known for certain, though it possibly works by creating a hostile environment for sperm (one patient observed that the sperm probably got tired 'looping the loop'!). It may also prevent implantation of the fertilised egg on to the wall of the uterus.

It is inserted by a doctor usually at the time of the period or just after. This makes for easier insertion and the woman is unlikely to be pregnant. It can be inserted just after an abortion, provided this has been done under sterile conditions. It can also be fitted four weeks after a birth, though not after a caesarean birth, when fitting must be delayed for three months so that the scar is properly healed. Insertion takes a few minutes and may cause slight bleeding and cramp-like pain. It should not be inserted if infection is present. Women are taught to check that the device is present by feeling the threads which hang in the vagina. If they can feel a 'hard' bit they are advised to return to the clinic or doctor as the coil is being extruded. The plastic-only coils do not need changing or renewing, though some doctors advocate a change after a certain number of years as the coil may become misshapen and encrusted with salts. The copper coils, however, do need changing after two years because they are no longer effective as a contraceptive. While any of the coils can be used by women who have had children the copper coils are used in women who have not had a baby, as they are smaller, easier to insert and have less chance of being expelled. The success of the coil depends on careful selection of the women, and the skill of the doctor. There is no evidence that the coil predisposes to cancer of the cervix or uterus.

It is contra-indicated where there is active pelvic infection, heavy prolonged periods or the possible presence of pregnancy.

Advantages It is reliable and convenient. Should the woman become pregnant with the coil *in situ* there is no risk of malformation to the child, although she may miscarry. Once the device is inserted, it is safe to have intercourse. When it is removed fertility returns.

Disadvantages It needs medical advice and help. It can cause heavy painful periods and so is not suitable for all women. If the periods are too heavy or frequent over the course of six months, it will have to be removed. It can be expelled out of the uterus; 50 per cent of all expulsions occur in the first year. Vaginal discharge can be increased, and this worries some women. It may perforate the uterus. It is occasionally difficult to remove. About 2 per cent of women may develop mild pelvic infections with the coil. These can be treated with antibiotics with the coil left in place. Most cases of infection are due to recurrence of an old infection. If pregnancy does occur with the coil inside the uterus it is advised that the coil be removed because of the risk of pelvic infection if the woman wants the pregnancy to continue.

Effectiveness 2–3 pregnancies per 100 women years. Pregnancy may occur with the device in place or with unnoticed expulsion. 5 per cent of pregnancies with the coil in place occur in the tube (ectopic pregnancy; 0.3 per cent of all pregnancies are ectopic). Pregnancy is more likely in the first few months of use.

Number of users of different methods, 1976

FPA Fact Sheet No. 31 (1976) gave the following rough estimates of the number of people using each method.

Oral contraceptive	3,000,000
The sheath	2,500,000
Coitus interruptus	1,400,000
The coil (IUD)	500,000
Rhythm method	400,000
The cap and cream	250,000
Chemicals alone	150,000

It is calculated that there are nearly 10½ million women in the fertile age range, of which 8 million are likely to be sexually active and at risk of pregnancy. Of these approximately 3 million women (or their partners) are *not* using any reliable form of contraception or are not using one regularly.

During the late 1960s studies revealed that the sheath, the pill and withdrawal were the most commonly used methods (Cartwright 1970, Woolf 1972, Bone 1973). By the mid-1970s it would appear that for all ages up to thirty-four years the pill is by far the most used method, followed by the sheath. In women over thirty-five years the sheath was the most used followed by withdrawal and the pill (Bone 1978). In young people (16—19 years) the sheath, the pill and withdrawal are the most commonly used methods (Farrell 1978).

Male Sterilisation: Vasectomy

This has become an increasingly popular method of birth control when the couple have decided that their family is complete. In the domiciliary setting it tends to be chosen by couples where the man has taken the responsibility for birth control by using the sheath or practising withdrawal.

The operation is simple and straightforward and is usually done under local anaesthetic, taking about 15 minutes on an outpatient basis. The vasa deferentia (the tubes carrying the sperms from the testicles to the seminal vesicles) are cut, a small piece (1—4 cm.) is removed and the ends are tied. The man is left with a small scar in the scrotum. He can be back at work the next day, provided he does not do heavy lifting for two weeks. This is to prevent the wound re-opening. The man may get swelling and bruising of the testicles. Some men say it feels as if they have had a kick in the scrotum and feel sore for a few days. Intercourse can be resumed whenever the couple wish, but other contraceptive precautions have to be taken until the semen is clear of the sperms which have been stored in the seminal vesicles. About 2—3 months after the operation the semen is examined and if two consecutive specimens are free of sperm then the man is told he can dispense with contraception. Ejaculation takes place in the normal way and neither sexual satisfaction nor potency is altered in any way. Sperms continue to be made but get re-absorbed so that the testes do not swell.

Counselling is advisable for any couple thinking of sterilisation, whether male or female. The consent of both is needed for either operation. In the case of vasectomy the man needs to know what is to be done, when he will be safe to dispense with other contraceptive precautions, that the operation does not affect the testicles or their functioning (they still release testosterone, the male hormone, and manufacture sperm, but these get absorbed), that there is minimal reduction in the volume of the ejaculate and that sex will feel the same without any alteration of potency. Other factors that need to be taken into account when counselling:

a) the health of the wife (for example she may have a gynaecological complaint that might require hysterectomy);

    b) the relationship of the couple — its stability;

    c) whether one partner is putting pressure on the other to be sterilised;

    d) the health of the existing children;

    e) the sexual relationship.

Vasectomy is not a solution to sexual difficulties unless these are due to fear of pregnancy. One married couple in their twenties, both teachers with no children, requested vasectomy because the world was overpopulated. As they were both active Christians they wished to devote their lives to the service of God and felt children would prevent them doing this. When the woman came to be examined she was found to be still a virgin. Their embarrassment about sex had prevented them from complaining about this. The wife subsequently went on the pill and sterilisation was deferred until they had considered the implications further. A year later they still did not want children but the wife decided to remain on the pill. The marriage had meanwhile been consummated after therapy, with the wife being taught to stretch her vagina as described earlier.

Advantages It is effective, about 100 per cent reliable; very occasionally the vasa reunite and sperm may appear in the semen.

Disadvantages The operation must be regarded as irreversible, though a few surgeons have joined the tubes together. Although the sperm may appear normal in every respect some men with reunited vasa fail to fertilise their partners. It is postulated that in these cases the man may become immunised to his own sperm though there may be other explanations. Thus when counselling the couple must be faced with the possibility of their spouse dying or the children being killed and how they would feel about this. So often in such counselling couples *have* given this much thought. A remark that another child could *not* replace existing children is commonly heard. The success of reversal of male sterilisation can be measured by the appearance of mobile sperms (this occurs in 75 per cent of cases) or by a pregnancy (this occurs in 45 per cent of cases).

Female sterilisation

The operation consists of removing a portion of the fallopian tubes and tying the ends so that the eggs can no longer travel down the tubes. The operation should not of itself affect the woman in any way. It can be done forty-eight hours after a birth, at the same time as a caesarean operation or as a special procedure. Her periods should remain the same, though menstrual irregularities requiring hysterectomy have been noted in those women who have been sterilised who had five or more children (Muldoon 1972). A few women complain of putting on weight after sterilisation and blame the operation. It may be that the woman at a deep psychological level feels castrated (although her ovaries, which produce the female sex hormones, remain untouched) and over-eats to comfort herself. The operation can be done through an abdominal cut or by using a special instrument (the laparascope) passed through a small cut just below the navel to visualise the tubes which are then burnt. This technique requires the woman to be in hospital for three days only. A general anaesthetic is used.

The successful reconnecting of the tubes is a difficult procedure and depends on how the operation was performed. It is estimated that successful reconnecting occurs in 30 per cent of cases. Thus sterilisation in the woman must be entered into with the acceptance of irreversibility. Counselling is necessary, as with the male, and the same factors need to be taken into account. Again, associated gynaecological complaints may make hysterectomy advisable rather than sterilisation. Where the operation is essential for the woman's health it can be performed without the husband's consent. Ways of performing reversible sterilisation are constantly being explored.

Advantages It is effective and reliable. The woman should not experience any physical side effects.

Disadvantages It is irreversible. As with any operation, there is the risk of sudden death. Peel & Potts (1969) estimate a mortality rate of 1 in 5,000 operations.

As mentioned above, physical sequelae are unlikely but what of psychological sequelae? It is important to ascertain these for two reasons: (1) Couples are increasingly opting for sterilisation once their families are complete as a solution to their contraceptive problems. 11 per cent of women interviewed by Bone (1978) had either been sterilised themselves or their partner had. Over 73 per cent of the women with five or more children had been sterilised. (2) Sterilisation, being an irreversible procedure done sometimes when the couple are in their late twenties or early thirties, gives time for unforeseen changes to occur that may lead to regret, such as loss of a child or partner or breaking of a marriage. As sterilisation entails a loss of function or an attribute, it might be expected to be accompanied by mourning for that loss and a readjustment to a new and altered body image. Another important factor which might cause psychological disturbance is the degree to which a person's concept of himself/herself as male or female is bound up with the ability to produce children. Related to this is the feeling of some men and women that if they are failures as people then at least having babies is something they *can* do. This, of course, is not necessarily associated with adequate rearing and caring of children once they arrive.

One significant drawback to almost all the studies is that they relate to feelings *after* the operation. In almost no study is there an attempt to form a psychological assessment of the person before the operation. Thus they are retrospective studies and as such their findings may be invalidated. Suppose, for example, a high incidence of depression is encountered after the operation it may be assumed that this is due to the operation, but, it is possible that the person may have suffered from depression before it. The evidence of dissatisfaction and regret after sterilisation is said to vary from 0 to 40 per cent among published follow-ups (Peel & Potts 1969). In answer to a simple question such as 'Would you have the operation again?', 'Are you sorry that you were sterilised?', only 2—5 per cent report regret (Adams 1954, Jensen & Lester 1957, Chaset 1962). In the report of the Simon Population Trust (December 1969), of 1,000 vasectomy cases only two couples reported deterioration in general health. For many there is an improvement in their sexual life (Thompson & Baird 1968). Those who are most disturbed by sterilisation are the men or women who have a history of previous psychiatric disturbance (Johnson 1964, Sim 1973) or where the doctor has recommended sterilisation for medical reasons (Barglow & Eisner 1966, Barnes & Zuspan 1958).

It may be difficult for men to avoid equating vasectomy with castration (Ziegler *et al.* 1966). Only 10 men out of 82 who replied to an offer of help for those unhappy about their vasectomy indicated some psychological problems arising from the operation and half of these had previous psychological instability (Wolfers 1970). Women who have been sterilised may blame all their subsequent misfortune in life upon it (Barglow & Eisner 1966). Some women who perceive sterilisation as a loss of function may have fantasies of pregnancy for a few months post-operatively. These feelings need to be worked through. The social worker is often the most suitable person to help the woman do this.

A serious criticism of all these studies is that no attempt has been made to investigate the attitudes of couples to contraception, to sex and their own sexuality, and to the quality of their relationship and the value which children have for them.

Request for reversal Another way of assessing satisfaction is to ascertain the number of individuals who request reversal. One request in 1,000 vasectomies (0.1 per cent) has been quoted, which is fairly constant in all cultures (Deys 1976). In Britain the request usually follows divorce and is not related to the age of the man.

Of 103 women requesting reversal of sterilisation at the Hammersmith Hospital during 1975-76 the predominant reason for the request was remarriage. Many of the women had not used contraception adequately prior to sterilisation, and though some said they had been inadequately counselled the same number admitted they had pressurised the gynaecologist to sterilise them (Winston 1977). (Of 367 patients sterilised through the Haringey Domiciliary Service, 239 women and 128 men, during 1968-78, only 3 have requested reversal.)

To summarise, it is difficult to assess the psychological effects of sterilisation. To date the majority who have had it done seem satisfied, with few long-lasting sequelae, and are relieved that they are free from the risk of unwanted pregnancy. And though there will always be a few couples for whom the operation will be a mixed blessing, and an attempt should be made to reduce this number by counselling and selection, nevertheless, the benefits seem to outweigh the disadvantages. Finally, to quote K. L. Oldershaw (1976) — 'women suffering from recurrent episodes of depression or anxiety are unlikely to use contraception either regularly or efficiently and repeated unwanted pregnancies would certainly have a greater total adverse psychological and physical effect than sterilisation'.

ATTITUDES, BELIEFS AND MYTHS RELATED TO INDIVIDUAL BIRTH CONTROL METHODS

The acceptability of any method depends on several factors:
   a) motivation to use a method or any method;
   b) knowledge;

c) safety and health hazards;

d) aesthetic factors which are related to ease of use;

e) cost (this should not now be a problem since contraception is available through the National Health Service);

f) effectiveness;

g) availability and how the method is presented.

The better educated are able to read and evaluate what they read and are thus less likely to rely on hearsay and old wives' tales. It is a truism that the perfect method of birth control does not exist. The perfect method would be 100 per cent effective. It would have no side effects or health hazards, it would not interfere with future fertility, nor with the sex act and it would be cheap and easy to use and obtain. Most couples learn sooner or later to put up with side effects, or inconvenience, or both, of a method, sometimes regarding its use as the lesser of two evils, namely an unwanted pregnancy. Confidence in a method is inspired by a friend's good experience. The reverse is also true. How knowledgeable are people about contraception? Most people know that there are methods of birth control and can name some of them, but they may not know how they work, their reliability, and the risks, if any, to health. Only 15% of the women who used the safe period in Woolf's Study (1972) actually knew how it worked. Peel & Carr (1972) found that only 55 per cent thought they were adequately informed. In a study of lower socio-economic groups, though an admittedly small sample (Askham 1975), a relatively high proportion knew little about sex or birth control.

This lack of knowledge necessarily colours attitudes to birth control. Added to this and influencing attitudes is the often hazy knowledge that many people have about their bodies, their genitals and the process of conception itself. It is sometimes thought that the man 'lays the egg' in the woman during intercourse, while she merely provides nourishment for the baby (This, of course, was the view held in the Middle Ages.) Among West Indian men and women seen in Haringey, a common belief is that the woman 'discharges' semen like the man when she has an orgasm and that that is how conception occurs. The corollary of this belief is that if the woman stops herself having an orgasm she will not get pregnant. When men and women are aware that the woman produces an egg they may have the vaguest notion about when it occurs. Some may believe it occurs during menstruation, so if intercourse is avoided at that time all will be well. There are many myths connected with menstruation — that it is a process to get rid of bad blood and if the woman fails to have a 'good' heavy period then this blood will travel to her brain and give her headaches. This is a commonly held belief among West Indian women, which may be one reason why they often prefer the coil since it may result in heavy periods. Some women believe that if they miss a period it is because it is 'blocked up' inside (not that they are pregnant: this, of course, may be wishful thinking!). The belief that it is the man who 'lays the egg' in the woman or that it is the 'man's stuff' that makes the baby (West Indian men believe that they 'know' the exact moment of conception) makes the male methods of birth control more easily understood. The belief in the efficiency of withdrawal can be such that if the woman does get pregnant when this method is used, the man doubts his paternity. He may accuse her of being unfaithful 'It can't be mine because I was being careful'.

Since the sheath is often associated with 'illicit' sex or sex with prostitutes it often has an unsavoury reputation and women are disgusted by it. There is a strong fear that the sheath will come off and get 'lost inside' and the woman will have to have an operation to remove it (and hence everyone will know that you are having sex).

This is related to the almost complete ignorance that many women have about their bodies. Unfortunately, it has been culturally acceptable that women should be kept in ignorance about their bodies. 'Nice women' do not look at or touch their genitalia — that would be akin to masturbation, unacceptable and unnecessary in the female. It is, therefore, not surprising that women (and men for that matter) have many myths and fantasies about women's genitalia to the extent that many women in the lower socio-economic groups, who have no access to books and diagrams, believe that they have 'one opening down below' through which urine, faeces, baby and all come down. Hence their difficulty in touching or examining themselves or in using internal tampons, caps or spermicides. It is not unexpected therefore, that many women's groups in the States have deliberately set out to teach women about their bodies and how to examine their own genitalia. Since most women do not know what they look like inside they have no concept of how big the vagina is or that it can stretch, hence the frequently heard expression from women who have painful intercourse or who cannot use tampons that they are 'too small'. The reaction of many women to the cap is, 'Oh, that's

too big, it will never go in me', or 'How do you get that in?'
Some women have to be shown exactly where their vaginal
opening is, some couples believe that the penis enters the
uterus during intercourse, others that the uterus is a large sack
filling the abdomen, hence the amazement of many women
when they are shown the coil: 'Isn't it small?' When asked how
big they thought it was, they frequently reply, 'I thought it
was like a bed spring that you had to coil up inside'. No wonder
many women are terrified of it! Men too are afraid of it and
talk of putting their penises into a bed of thorns and complain
that the coil hurts them. This can have a realistic basis if the
coil is being extruded through the cervix, but in the majority
of cases it is the fear of being hurt and an over-active imagination that causes the pain. Other beliefs about the coil are that
if the woman gets pregnant with it inside, then the baby will be
deformed — the coil will get lodged in its brain. Some West
Indian girls believe that the coil causes venereal disease. This
notion probably arises because of the increased cervical secre-
tion of mucus that occurs with a coil.

The mechanical methods of birth control such as the cap or
the sheath require a purposeful action in relation to intercourse.
Since sex and intercourse is often considered to be a
spontaneous, impulsive act, couples may find that having to use
such a method puts them off intercourse altogether: it is too
premeditated. This tends to happen when couples do not know
each other well or are ambivalent about sex and their own
sexuality in particular. A couple confident about their sexuality
and their relationship and not afraid to anticipate the pleasure
of sex can often incorporate the using of such a method into
their love play. For example the woman can put the sheath on
her partner. There are other fears connected with the cap, apart
from those associated with actually inserting it. These are to do
with taking the sexual initiative. By putting the cap in before
they start to make love the woman may feel she is somehow
usurping the man's role and that she is being a 'bad woman'. If
the man is uncertain of his potency he may feel threatened by
his wife using the cap and taking the control of the contraception. However, if the woman does not put the cap in before love
play he may feel that she does not really want sex. Thus, if a
couple cannot discuss it openly with each other and joke about
it, the cap will be especially daunting to use. It is understandable that men find sex better without the sheath since it does
interfere with sensation, but the fact that it remains widely used

suggests that many men cope with it without too much difficulty, putting up with it perhaps because other methods are disliked even more. Some men, however, express anxieties that it might break or tear or that it might have a hole in it. These anxieties are often used as an excuse for not using the sheath for selfish reasons. Some men are explicit about their dislike — 'like going to bed with your wellingtons on', or 'using the sheath makes one less of a man' — and others are concerned about their potency with the sheath. One married man said he was 'allergic to them rubbers'. When questioned more closely about the allergy, he revealed that he lost his erection when he put a sheath on. It was suggested that his wife could do this for him. He thought women should not do that, and anyway his wife never touched his penis.

Attitudes to the mechanical methods for the very reason that these are intimately associated with intercourse often reveal the man's or woman's attitude to sex itself, which can be useful in diagnosing a sexual problem. In the family planning clinics teaching a woman how to use a cap often results in helping her to understand and accept her own vagina. Some women complain about the messiness of the cap since it must be used with spermicidal cream. However, this again may mean a rejection of the 'messiness' of sex. For some women the sheath is attractive because it protects them from the 'messiness' — that is the man's semen. They dislike the 'slime' and are over-obsessed with hygiene and cleanliness. Oral sex is anathema to them. They often form part of the clientele of gynaecological clinics with recurrent complaints about 'discharge' for which the doctor can find no cause. Men can be embarrassed to go in to a chemist to buy the sheath.

Pessaries are disliked for similar reasons to the cap because they are messy and because the woman needs to touch her genitals to use them.

The pill is probably the most widely known of all the contraceptive methods. Its popularity is the result of its ease of use, its effectiveness and because it is unrelated to the act of intercourse. The pill is often regarded as a powerful drug since it needs to be prescribed by a doctor. However, since doctors do prescribe it, it also gives reassurance ('doctor knows best'). The pill has suffered from a bad press and many attempts have been made to disparage it (as the sheath was disparaged in the past) — that it is used by 'loose' women, that it leads to promiscuity, that it means sex without the punishment, i.e. the baby, and that it has led to the rise in the venereal rate. Thus it provokes extreme reactions, from those who think that every girl should go on the pill as soon as she starts menstruation to those who believe it has caused the decline in morality. It is damned by its very virtues, namely its ease of use and efficiency. It makes sex too easy. Thus its side effects and risk to health are often exaggerated, particularly by the popular press. Women are the sufferers. Every time there is a new pill scare (and these occur with monotonous regularity) pills are thrown away, women become pregnant and then may want an abortion. This phenomenon has been seen several times, particularly among domiciliary family planning patients who are less able to evaluate the risks associated with the pill. Thus women are often afraid of the pill. They may resent it because it makes sex easy — 'If it wasn't for the pill I wouldn't have sex because I could tell my boyfriend I was scared to get pregnant'. The resentment is sometimes felt by married women too 'why should I take the risks when he gets all the pleasure?' This is particularly true of women who do not enjoy sex; they often produce symptoms so that the doctor tells them to stop taking it.

One of the most difficult problems connected with the pill lies in trying to find out just what is a genuine complaint as opposed to the feelings of ambivalence, fear and resentment that may magnify a trivial side effect but may not be admitted. Headaches are a frequent complaint when women are taking the pill; how far is this genuine or the result of tension associated with fear of taking the pill? Loss of libido is another case in point — 'the pill puts you off sex'. This again is very difficult to evaluate. Some women dislike the 100% effectiveness of the pill — they like taking chances. Others feel sex is only right when there is the possibility of getting pregnant, since sex is basically for procreation. This is not to say that women do not have genuine complaints and side effects with the pill, but to illustrate how difficult these are to evaluate and that complaints may not be as straightforward as they seem.

see p. 151

There are many mistaken ideas on the risks of taking the pill. Some women believe it is fatal to take it — they will be the 'unlucky ones'. Taking a pill every day seems 'unnatural'. With both 'medical' methods, the pill and the coil, there is the anxiety of being controlled by outside forces. For a few couples birth control itself is considered 'unnatural', much as the medical profession thought it was unphysiological seventy years ago. Some women may feel unable to be responsible for themselves, so reject the pill or the cap and look for 'outer control' by requesting the coil or sterilisation.

Sterilisation both for men and women is a final step and thus many fears and myths are attached to it. There is a common belief that sex will be no good afterwards and that the person who has been sterilised will not be attractive to his or her partner. Sterilisation is sometimes equated with loss of virility and femininity. Men fear they will become impotent, that ejaculation will not take place in the usual way, or at all. Women think they will become like a 'spayed cat' and will get fat and lazy. Some women believe that sterilisation means 'taking everything away', including the uterus, tubes and ovaries.

12

Contraceptive Counselling

Contraceptive counselling is a term usually applied to discussions held between a doctor, nurse or social worker and a
woman or couple, in a clinic setting (family planning, post-
natal, post-abortion). Domiciliary family planning, that is giving
advice in the home, is a specialised form of contraceptive
counselling. It will be looked at separately. Contraceptive
counselling can also be used to apply to the more difficult
situation that exists in the home where discussions on family
planning take place between a social worker or health visitor
and a woman (or couple), though a method is not actually
prescribed.

CONTRACEPTIVE COUNSELLING IN THE CLINIC

The clinic procedure has already been described. The woman
attending a family planning clinic has usually both accepted the
idea of family planning and chosen a method (commonly the
pill). Provided that there are no medical contra-indications, all
that is needed is information, examination and teaching. It has
been noted in Part 1 that the vaginal examination can reveal
sexual difficulties which cannot consciously be admitted and
there may be a need for further counselling.

The choice of method

This can reveal much about the relationship, attitudes to sex,
the body and the woman's own sexuality. Thus when the
woman chooses the method it may be because she wants to be
in control and cannot rely on her partner. Choosing the pill or
coil rather than the cap may mean that she wants a very reliable
method. Alternatively, it may mean that she does not want to
be involved in the messiness of sex or her own body. Choosing
less reliable methods such as the safe period or chemicals may

indicate that the woman has sex infrequently and sees no point in taking the pill regularly, or it could mean that subconsciously she really wants to be pregnant. If the man chooses the sheath (rare at family planning clinics) then it may be because he wishes to be in control, is afraid of the health hazards associated with the female methods, or is afraid that his partner will be unfaithful.

Complaints about methods

These may have a realistic basis or they may reflect a crisis in the relationship, a covert wish to get pregnant, sexual difficulties or general discontent with domestic circumstances (money, housing, the children) which cannot be expressed consciously. Loss of interest in sex with the pill often falls into this category. One young married woman with a child of three complained at a family planning clinic that she had no interest in sex and blamed the pill. Since she looked depressed this was not accepted at face value. On further discussion it emerged that she was lonely and bored at home and missed her friends at work. She was also worried about her attitude to her daughter. She resented her and feared she might harm her. The complaint disappeared when she got a part-time job, leaving the child to go in a nursery while she worked. She is still taking the pill.

Requests to change methods, or stopping a method when pregnancy is not really intended, also come into this category. Unless the underlying problems are revealed and helped, persuasion to choose a method or stay on a method will only be a temporary solution. The woman may well fail to keep subsequent appointments. This may be one possible explanation for the drop-out rate from clinics, which is stated to be as high as 30 per cent (Ward 1971). Should the woman become pregnant in these circumstances the stress may be very great. Feelings of regret, confusion, guilt about getting pregnant may be worsened by the solution she chooses (abortion, adoption or keeping the child), especially if she is also rejected by the partner.

CONTRACEPTIVE COUNSELLING OUTSIDE THE CLINIC
The role of the social worker

In many ways the role of the social worker in family planning is more difficult than that of other professional workers, such as health visitors and doctors. This may be one explanation of the reluctance of social workers to become involved in family planning. Although tacit approval is given towards the idea of family planning, little practical action may be taken. Allen (1974) found that although social workers as a group were most in favour of a family planning campaign and the setting up of domiciliary services, they were probably the group that did the least. An unpublished dissertation (Mortimer 1971) showed the reluctance of probation officers to discuss family planning or refer clients to clinics. Many probation officers did not know where their local clinics were situated.

Reference has already been made to another possible explanation of the reluctance to be involved, viz. very little programmed teaching or social work courses about either sexuality or contraception. There are, of course, other issues that face the social worker in relation to family planning which may be at variance with the philosophical concepts and ideals of social work practice and these may form the true basis for the reluctance of the social worker to be involved in family planning and sexual problems. There are perhaps two main schools of thought in social work practice — the older (historically) casework approach (which has its roots in psychoanalysis) and the socio-political approach. According to the first school, it is the client and his maladaptation who is seen to be the problem. The social worker's role here is to clarify exactly what the problem is and help the client to develop insight into the ways in which his own behaviour contributes to or exacerbates his difficulties. This is done in a non-directive way. Opponents of this approach argue that this is merely helping the client to adjust to the *status quo* and that it is this that needs changing. Hence the second approach to social work, which concerns itself with the client's environment. The argument runs that by changing this, that is by improving housing, making more and better paid jobs available, having better schools and so on, the client will be helped to function more adequately as an individual. It is possible that the majority of social workers use a mixture of the two approaches to help clients with problems. Both these approaches in their extreme forms have found themselves at odds with the idea of discussing family planning with the client. If casework is being done, then discussion of family planning might seem as if the social worker is being directive and telling the client what to do, which is contrary to the theory and practice of casework and an invasion of the client's privacy.

Hence the anxiety to maintain client self-determination. With the second approach the need for improved social conditions is seen to be crucial to helping the poor. Family planning is seen as making only a minor and insignificant contribution. There is also the anxiety that family planning will be exploited by government as the solution to all social ills, ignoring the need for expenditure on housing, schools and so on.

To the client who is seeking social work help with, for example, housing or financial problems, discussion about family size or family planning may seem either irrelevant or an interference with private concerns.

The social worker is more likely to be involved with those who are ambivalent or hostile to the idea of family planning. The woman may have failed to attend a clinic or GP for advice or only attended a few times and her partner may refuse to practise withdrawal or use the sheath. Since it may be a question of motivation and persuasion, each social worker will have to define his own role and position. In connection with this, social workers (as with other carers) will need to be aware of how far their own attitudes to contraception can influence those of their clients. The 'iatrogenic' cause of ineffective or non-use of contraception — that is, caused by the negative or ambivalent attitudes of the professional — has been noted by Sandberg & Jacobs (1971). These feelings may be derived from the professional person's own guilt and anxiety about sex and contraception. Equally, authoritarian, over-enthusiastic and dogmatic attitudes about contraception or a particular method on the part of the professional adviser can lead to suspicion, resentment and ultimately refusal of both the adviser and the method. Thus the social worker will have to tread a careful path between the two. The choices open to social workers in relation to contraception are as follows:

(1) To provide information only in response to a request for it. The social worker may be misled into thinking that because few ask then few really want to know. The client may perceive that the social worker is not comfortable about sexual matters and decides not to ask. (This is similar to the GPs telling Cartwright (1970) that they only gave information when requested; but, as she stated, women *want* the professional worker to initiate discussions. This then gives them the freedom to speak.)

(2) To make a referral again only in response to a request, the same kind of barriers in communication, the burden of

initiating discussions, being placed on the client again.

(3) To initiate discussion, explore areas of conflict, clear up misinformation, give information and make the necessary referrals and arrangements where appropriate. This might mean actually taking a client to the clinic or referring to an agency such as the domiciliary service.

Thus the role of the social worker in family planning, as in other areas of his work, can be that of educator, facilitator and enabler. The social worker, by being concerned about this aspect of the client's life, can help the client realise and appreciate its importance.

In order to initiate discussion the social worker must be clear about his aims and what he hopes to achieve. He must also be properly informed and reasonably comfortable about sex and family planning. This is encouraging for the client and allows freer expression of feelings and needs and also, of course, it will give sanction to sexual activity and pleasure. Comfort does not imply that the social worker should not have moral standards with regard to sex. He may also be involved in making value judgements. This should not occasion anxiety provided that these judgements are held in awareness and are above board and not imposed. Comfort comes with practice and first attempts may well be mishandled. Part of the comfort with sex is related to sexual language. Clients may well be ashamed and embarrassed that they do not know the 'correct' words. It is not recommended that the professional goes in for four-letter words with the client (who may well be embarrassed for the professional worker who does use them) but it is essential for both to understand what is being said and to convey to the couple that they are understood. The class/cultural differences in the use of sexual words has already been noted.

Discussion about birth control often provides a unique opportunity for doing some straightforward sex education in its widest sense about the body, reproduction and the sexual response. This is particularly helpful for mothers with young children.

Initiating discussion on birth control may be more difficult in some ways for the social worker than for other professionals (bearing in mind that they, too, had and have difficulties); in other ways it may be easier. For example, when a social and family history is being taken and questions asked about pregnancies and their outcome the client can be asked, 'Did you plan it that way?' Some clients may be surprised, but provided questions are asked in a gentle, non-judgemental way, most will be grateful for being given an opportunity to discuss this area of their lives. Awareness of any conflicts within the relationship or marriage can also form a basis for discussion about sexual difficulties and family planning. Sometimes it may be the method itself that is interfering with the sexual relationship, or it may alter the dominant/submissive role relationship between husband and wife and this in turn may lead to marital difficulties.

Sometimes a couple may feel that another child will patch up a marriage. Again this provides an opportunity for the social worker to explore past behaviour, particularly related to family planning, and to see whether this solution is really likely to be effective.

When the behaviour of the child leads to the involvement of the social services, a question such as 'Did you go in for him/her?' can be used to open up the subject of contraception and allow attitudes to it to be explored.

Illness and stress (from whatever cause) within the family may make it vital for the mother's health for her not to become pregnant for a time. Mothers with two or more children under five confined to flats are often under great stress. The social worker can focus the discussion on the need for spacing of children so that the mother can have a rest, and again this enables the subject of contraception to be raised.

In connection with stress, as in the case of the family in which non-accidental injury to children has occurred, contraception and the need for child spacing may need to be urgently explored. However, such parents often have a negative attitude to family planning (Smith 1975). The social worker may need to explore these attitudes through the relationship, including the sexual relationship, of the couple.

Complaints about the methods or statements such as 'My doctor says I cannot take the pill, use the coil etc.' should not deter the social worker because the woman may really be saying 'I don't like sex and I don't see why I should put up with the risks of the pill/coil'. The need to use the fear of pregnancy to control the amount of sexual activity may also be relevant. Similarly, statements such as 'My husband does not want me to take the pill/have the coil', should not be accepted at face value. They may serve to mask the woman's own fears and anxieties.

The stopping of a method (particularly by the woman) where

a pregnancy is not consciously intended should occasion concern. The relationship may be breaking up and the woman's refusal to persist with contraception may be her way of saying to the partner, 'I refuse to have sex with you'. Unfortunately, the partner usually ignores this and the woman may well be left with an unwanted pregnancy.

Ambivalence about starting or persevering with a method of contraception will need exploration. There may be fear of contraception harming fertility or health or a fear of being controlled. There may be doubts about the relationship or another pregnancy. The ambivalence may be due to cultural and religious factors.

Referral

The successful uptake of family planning may well depend on how well the referral has been made. Thus the social worker will need to familiarise himself with the local clinics and get to know the staff so that direct referral can be made. The client should also be prepared for the experience. The detail with which this is done needs to be gauged for each client. Too much or too little detail can cause unnecessary anxiety.

Fear of the internal (the vaginal examination) may deter some women (particularly those belonging to lower socio-economic groups) from going to a clinic. There may be fantasies of being ripped and torn by the vaginal speculum, known colloquially as the shoe horn. The fears may be related to unpleasant experiences of being examined in labour. The woman may also fear it because she feels it may reveal something about her sexuality that she wishes to keep hidden or deny — that she really is a sexual woman and enjoys sex.

The social worker will need to decide whether merely informing the woman about local clinics is enough or whether the woman should be taken to the clinic or whether referral to a domiciliary service should be made. This decision will be influenced by the knowledge the social worker has of the client's ability to use sources of help and the extent to which she has availed herself of them in the past. It may be that fear, embarrassment etc. have been the main barriers in attending a clinic. In other cases situational factors may have been the main obstacles, such as inaccessibility of the clinic, awkward times, small children to care for and so on. It may be that the woman or couple are poorly motivated to use contraception.

Difficulties with motivation

When a woman (or couple) is reluctant or refuses to use contraception even though it would be in her own or her family's best interests the social worker will need to decide what to do about this. This is obviously a delicate and controversial issue since it entails a value judgement about what are the women's best interests and the individual's right to choose. Should the social worker decide not to interfere the consequences could be disastrous with, for example, another child at risk from non-accidental injury. If the social worker does attempt to motivate the woman to use contraception then he runs the risk of provoking hostility. This may either make any future work very difficult or prevent it altogether. However, similar issues arise over the decision to take a child into care. A value judgement is made about parental capability to care adequately for the child. Removing the child often provokes great anger and hostility which has to be worked through.

Often the hostility to family planning is more apparent than real since it is bound up with fears and anxieties about sex, the contraceptive methods and the services offering advice already examined. Allied to this, the couple may never have really discussed sex or their feelings and needs and how many children they want and can realistically cope with (both emotionally and financially) and hence pregnancies just 'happen'. This can lead to fatalistic attitudes about contraception actually working. The social worker by being relaxed and open can create a secure environment for sharing these difficulties.

However, there may be deeper-seated causes for the hostility not only to the contraceptive methods but to the idea of controlling fertility. These may have to do with the individual and/ or the relationship. They are often due to faulty parenting — feelings of rejection and worthlessness allied to difficulties in making or sustaining satisfying and fulfilling relationships. Immaturity and difficulty in learning from life's experiences are associated factors. The ability to become pregnant, pregnancy itself and children may then become the principal concerns of a person's life, overriding and dominating everything else. Thus some very deprived women only feel 'full' when they are pregnant. The woman may see no other role for herself than that of mother. The concept of motherhood may be a limited one confined to being pregnant and the care of small babies — the baby being an extension of the woman herself.

Such women often find it hard to relate to the growing child or to take pleasure from its development. They feel excluded by the child's independence. One mother of five, when asked why she wanted another baby, expressed these feelings by saying, 'Well the youngest doesn't need me any more, he can walk and talk'. He was four years old. If these mothers are sterilised they may try to prolong the babyhood of the youngest.

For other women (and couples) children are used as a means to an end — status symbols of adulthood, femininity and virility. Parents who feel impotent and insecure in the adult world may use their children to parent them and form bulwarks against the outside world: These children are often kept home deliberately from school. This condition is often associated with agoraphobia and paranoid ideas about neighbours. Children are then used to do all the shopping and vet callers at the door. Disappointment with children in terms of appearance or behaviour may lead to rejection and further pregnancies to replace them.

For some couples another baby is the only 'new' thing in their life, creating interest, excitement and hope for the future. For some teenage girls a baby may be seen in a similar way rather like a new toy or novelty. Men who feel ineffectual outside the home may usurp the mother's role with the children; the mother may then have further pregnancies to fulfil her own needs. Some men feel that the only way to control a woman and at the same time deter rivals is to impregnate her repeatedly. Such men tend to be hostile to family planning and refuse to allow the woman to use contraception. Yet other men may see the woman only in the role of mother and provided she is busy with the children she will not make demands on him. Thus he will be free to pursue his own interests. A poor relationship between the man and woman may lead both to turn towards their children for emotional warmth and support. There are, and can be, no simple or quick solutions to these problems. The social worker will have to rely on the relationship he builds with the couple or the woman to serve as a model for care and trust, which can then be used to strengthen the couple's relationship and enable them to form relationships outside the family. Sometimes practical solutions such as involvement in community centres or helping the man and woman to obtain work may increase their sense of self-importance and worth and frees them from the extreme dependence on their children.

Shared care of the client

The social worker will often need to work in conjunction with family planning personnel belonging to a clinic or domiciliary service. For those families in need of special care with contraception the team approach may be essential. As with any shared care, there is a need for professional trust and respect. Stereotyped views of doctors and nurses (and vice versa) need to be guarded against. Close and frequent liaison may be necessary for effective work to be done. The client needs to be aware of this. There are a number of hazards with shared care, not least being those concerned with professional jealousy and rivalry, uncertainty about boundaries and responsibilities, and the client manipulating one worker against another.

A family planning service which shares many of the characteristics of field social work is the domiciliary family planning service. It can be used by the social worker to provide more intensive care with family planning.

Community work

Although the two main approaches to social work (casework and trying to effect changes socio-politically) have been examined earlier, there is, of course, a third approach, that of getting a community to draw on its own resources and help itself. This can also be used in family planning. A social worker working at a community centre helped to organise mothers' groups. Some meetings consisted of informal chats, others had an invited speaker to address the group on topics suggested by the mothers themselves or the social worker. One suggestion made by the social worker was to invite a speaker on family planning. The mothers were enthusiastic and the meeting was very lively with the mothers having an opportunity to discuss all the old wives' tales and anxieties about the pill, coil and sterilisation. Many admitted they were taking the pill and discussed their experiences with it and their treatment by clinics and doctors (some unflattering comments were made about both). Older women talked about their husbands having a vasectomy and this helped to clear up many misunderstandings.

One of the residential workers at a children's home contacted her local family planning clinic and asked if the doctor could come and speak to the children of both sexes, whose ages ranged from 13 to 16. She suspected that a few had had intercourse and others were 'on the brink'. The children, many of whom came from desperately deprived backgrounds, were very lively and eager to question and learn.

These are just two examples of the ways in which the community can be involved in discussions about family planning. Youth clubs, remand homes, approved schools and prisons are other settings for such discussions. A family planning speaker (FPA trained) has for the last few years been involved in talking to groups of boys in approved schools in the West Country. Several of these, unbeknown to the authorities in charge of them, were unmarried fathers.

Thus many possibilities are available to social workers, whether in the community or in a residential home, to play a constructive role in the field of family planning. They are in the unique position of being able to provide informed help, which can be tailored to suit the individual client's needs.

DOMICILIARY FAMILY PLANNING SERVICES

Domiciliary family planning services were set up initially as pilot projects in the late 1950s in Newcastle, York and Southampton. Their aim was to help the 'hard to reach' — the women who could not or would not go to clinics. These women usually belonged to social classes IV and V. The success of these projects (Peberdy & Morgans 1965, Mitchell 1967), made even more remarkable in that the only methods then available were the sheath, the cap and spermicides, led other local authorities to set up domiciliary services. There were about 140 in Britain, though this number has been reduced to about 50 (FPA personal communication).

The structure and function of the services

They are usually run by female staff — 1—2 doctors and several (1—6) nurses, all family-planning-trained. The Glasgow service (Wilson 1978), one of the largest, has 7 doctors and 10 nurses working part-time. The staff tend to be self-selected, seeing a need that can only be met by home visiting. They are usually prepared for the unpredictable, which goes with such work outside the structured clinic setting. The work requires patience, adaptability and an ability to cope with frustration and on rare occasions hostility.

The services rely on referral of cases from local services such as area social work teams, health visitors, hospital doctors, nurses, GPs and midwives. Thus it is important that the referring agents recognise the needy cases and present the domiciliary services in a constructive and positive way. The more successful services in terms of acceptability to the community have a large proportion of self-referred cases.

The procedure in the home is similar to that already described in the clinic setting. However, in domiciliary family planning work there is greater emphasis on psychosocial aspects. The initial visit, usually made by the doctor, is crucial in several respects, firstly, in establishing contact and enabling the woman to see what the service has to offer, and secondly, in allowing a comprehensive history to be taken covering varying aspects of the woman's life, not just the medical and obstetric ones. In particular some assessment needs to be made of the quality and stability of her relationships (past and present) with her parents, her partner and her children and the degree of motivation to use contraception. Although a complete picture of the woman and her life-style cannot be gained in one interview, it should reveal which areas need further exploration. It should also give some indication of the amount of support that the woman will need.

After a full discussion about methods the woman is asked which she prefers. It is essential that the woman chooses the method, provided there are no medical contra-indications. If the pill is chosen, packets are marked with the dates to start and stop and given to her. A vaginal examination is done. However, this is not insisted upon if the woman objects, though the reasons for this are explored. Some services fit coils at home, others prefer to arrange transport to clinics. Caps are rarely chosen for reasons already described, namely, the need for privacy and comfort with one's body. Sheaths and pessaries can be posted regularly when these are chosen (they are usually chosen by stable married couples). Sterilisation (male and female) can be arranged with prior counselling of the couple at home. Counselling can be provided for the unwanted pregnancy and referral for abortion arranged if this is requested. Psychosexual counselling for sexual difficulties can also be given. The domiciliary nurses usually do the subsequent follow-up visits every few weeks or months, depending on the woman's needs, involving the doctor where necessary. The domiciliary team keep in close contact about cases and support each other. This is essential since some of the families visited have great emotional needs and can be both demanding and manipulative. The domiciliary workers need to understand just what kind of transaction is taking place between themselves and the woman and why they find some women or situations more difficult to cope with than others. For example, if the woman is always out when the worker calls, various explanations are possible. The woman could be angry with the worker, ambivalent about continuing with contraception, or testing whether the worker is really concerned.

This is especially relevant to some depressed women. Their past and present experience of significant people in their lives (parents, sexual, marital partner) may be one of inconsistency and unreliability. This conditions their expectations of any professional helper — that they too will let them down, hence the need to test this out.

Complaints about methods, requesting a change of method or stopping a method where pregnancy is not intended have the same causes as already discussed. They need careful investigation. When life is unpredictable anyway, it is easy to abandon a method and risk pregnancy and then blame fate or God or say it was 'just one of those things'. The woman (or couple) needs to be helped to take the full responsibility for her own actions and their consequences. This necessary step in growing up may not have been fully accomplished. For some couples the fact that a method works can be very threatening since it implies that other areas of their lives might also be controlled. Some women in this situation deliberately forget pills or pull coils out and then allow fate to take a hand. Again help is necessary to enable the woman to understand her need to behave in this way.

The success of the domiciliary service in terms of client responsibility and perseverance with contraception depends partly on the staff's reliability. This is aided by the low turnover of domiciliary staff noted by Allen (1976). Once a trusting relationship has been established (the time taken to achieve this is obviously variable) it can serve as an alternative model of 'caring and mothering' that is not bound up solely with pregnancy and the having of babies but rather provides attention and care to the individual, namely the mother herself. The domiciliary staff are often put into the 'good parent' role and the woman will take the pill, for example, for the good parent. Of course, erratic use of a method and behaving like a naughty child can be used to test the 'parents' and see how they respond to 'naughty' behaviour. After some time, which may take months or years, the woman herself will take the responsibility for contraception. She may show this by telling the staff not to mark up packets of pills, or she may request transfer to the clinic. However, some women may never reach this stage and need continuing support. Alternatively, they may request sterilisation so that they no longer have to be responsible.

Once the woman is satisfactorily established on a method she can be transferred to the clinic or GP, whichever she prefers. Both the GP and referring agent are informed about the domiciliary visit and the method chosen. Liaising with other services and attending case conferences, where appropriate, is (or should be) an integral part of domiciliary work. Although couples are seen by the service, it is usually the woman who has most contact. The woman is given the doctor's and nurses' phone numbers so that problems can be sorted out as they arise, e.g. with a method or suspected pregnancy. This enables confidence to be built up in both the method chosen and the domiciliary service. One of the main advantages of a domiciliary service is the speed with which decisions can be taken and implemented. This is vital when dealing with families that are highly mobile and where domestic crises are a frequent occurrence.

The families that can best be helped by domiciliary family planning are those discussed in Chapter 13.

Some views on domiciliary services

The positive part that can be played by domiciliary services in family planning have been noted by several writers (Rainwater 1965, Cartwright 1970, Askham 1975). Others, notably Allen (1976), have been highly critical and feel there is a very limited need for such services. The domiciliary services are often accused of creating dependence and of not seeing the 'right', i.e. most needy, families. However, these same needy families are very likely to be involved with the social services that seem to experience most difficulty in referring cases (Allen 1974, Christopher 1975, Wilson 1978). Thus it is perhaps not surprising that not all the most needy cases are visited. General practitioners on the whole have similar negative attitudes, seeing domiciliary services as 'necessary only for those of very low intelligence or who are psychiatrically disturbed and who have refused the offer of sterilisation or an IUD' (Oldershaw 1976). Setting aside the obvious need of those who are too physically or mentally handicapped to use a clinic and those with language difficulties, these negative views ignore two significant points.

(1) Although possibly few in number, relative to the rest of the population, there *are* women or couples who do have special problems with contraception, as regards both motivation and perseverance in use. The consequences of further pregnancies may well be disastrous both for themselves and for their existing children.

(2) The short-sighted view of family planning is to see it merely as writing out a prescription or fitting a device. This may be all that is needed for the highly motivated woman who knows what she wants. However, much more is needed for those who are ambivalent about contraception, uncertain about themselves and their relationships and have poor or limited future prospects. Initiating the use of a method *is* an important part of family planning, but pills can be stopped and coils pulled out the following day or week. It is the *sustained* use that is the most vital aspect of family planning — the integration of contraception as an accepted part of a person's life.

Thus the domiciliary service is not merely or only a glorified postal service (though it may be just that for couples whose barriers to contraception use are physical rather than emotional) or a way of spoonfeeding the 'feckless and inadequate'. It should be a means of enabling the poorly motivated woman or couple to appreciate the significance and value of family planning not only for themselves and their relationships but also for their families. This is what takes time, practice and skill. If a domiciliary service is functioning properly it should be seeing only those in most need. This, in turn, depends on agencies such as social services recognising and referring such cases.

Thus the two main advantages of domiciliary family planning are:

a) to provide an opportunity for discussion in the privacy of a woman's home;

b) to provide continuing support for women who are

i) poorly motivated to persevere with contraception either through their own psychological problems or through relationship/marriage problems, and

ii) highly mobile.

The way domiciliary services function, working as they do in the grey area between medicine and social work and incorporating features of both, should make them an ideal agency for use by the social services. It is unfortunate that domiciliary services have not made more widely known what they do and what they can achieve.

The following case, an example of 'shared care' taken from the Haringey domiciliary service, was referred by a social worker. It illustrates the enormous amount of support over a considerable period of time that some families need.

Case history: Mrs W.

Mrs W. was referred for domiciliary family planning after the birth of her fourth child. She had failed several clinic appointments. She was twenty-three years old and had had four children in five years. She had been pregnant before marriage. This latest child was unwanted. The family were in considerable debt though the husband, a carpenter, was in regular work. Mrs W. would abandon the children from time to time. She had taken the pill erratically in the past but stopped because of side effects.

At the first visit by the domiciliary service she gave the impression of someone without any cares. She apologised for the state of the place (which was very dirty), something she was to do repeatedly on subsequent occasions. The children were half-clothed. She decided to take the pill. The nurse did the follow-up visits every two months for the first year. During that time there were numerous complaints (nausea, weight problems, depression) about the pill and it was changed twice with no improvement. She had also moved to another address, owing to debts. When the baby was a year old she left the children for a month, blaming the pill and saying it made her depressed. Significantly, her social worker had left and a new one took over at this time. Contact was difficult to maintain. Eventually she was located and she was still taking the pill. It was obvious that she missed her first social worker and had idealised her. She made various derogatory remarks about the new worker. The doctor responded to this by saying it took time to get used to a new person and that she must feel sad about the other one leaving. Mrs W. cried in response to this but said nothing.

Two months later she left again and the baby, now fifteen months old, had to be taken into care during her absence. Contact was maintained between the domiciliary service and the social worker. When Mrs W. did return she told the social worker she feared she was pregnant. The domiciliary doctor visited and confirmed the pregnancy. At this visit Mrs W. was sad and tearful, blaming herself. She said she always tried to be clean and tidy. The doctor interpreted this as referring to herself and keeping her own life clean and tidy. At this Mrs W. cried and said the pregnancy was not her husband's and that he came from a better family than she did. Her mother, who was always leaving home, finally left when she was eleven and she and her seven brothers and sisters had to be taken into care. There were further tears as the doctor expressed concern about this and Mrs W. said she could not go through with the pregnancy and wanted an abortion. This was arranged.

After the abortion, arrangements were made for her to have a coil. She failed to keep the appointment (was out when the nurse called to take her) and another visit was made by the doctor. This time the husband was there. He said little and appeared long-suffering. Mrs W. talked more about her mother — how she liked a gay time and had many men friends and had deceived the father who was described as strict and hardworking. She recalled an incident when her mother attempted to procure an abortion on herself with soap and water. This seemed an obvious reference to her own abortion and perhaps a need to be punished. She was asked about the abortion. She had expected it to be painful. She then talked about her youngest child, how she wanted him back but felt she could not cope. Contraception was then discussed. She was afraid of the coil and the pill was too much bother. Her husband wanted a vasectomy though she was concerned he might want more children. He denied this and said she had been through enough and he would have something done. Discussion between the doctor and social worker later revealed similar shared anxieties about this decision and possible regrets, particularly by Mrs W. who might want further children. The social worker remarked that Mr W. behaved like a doormat and always took Mrs W. back (rather like Mrs. W's father). Perhaps by deciding to have a vasectomy he was attempting to assert himself. The vasectomy was done at Mr W.'s insistence, despite these misgivings. The case was then closed by the domiciliary service.

A year later Mrs W. recontacted the domiciliary service. She had left her husband and was five months pregnant. The youngest child was now in care. She had a new boyfriend much younger than herself who was 'good' to her. She was ashamed to tell the social worker about the pregnancy. She could not have an abortion as her boyfriend would leave her. She would be sterilised after this pregnancy. She was reassured that no one would force her to have an abortion and was advised to tell her social worker the truth. (The fears about being made to have an abortion were related to the guilt she felt about having one child still in care.) She had had no ante-natal care as a result of her unsettled existence and the need to keep the pregnancy secret. The baby was born prematurely and had to be kept in hospital. Mrs W. took her own discharge after three days without being sterilised. The social worker, concerned about her attitude to the baby, discussed the possibility of adoption. A home visit by the doctor revealed a marked contrast in Mrs W. The new home was spotlessly clean and Mrs W. looked well. This was commented upon. She said she felt happier and was trying to keep a nice place for her older children (aged nine, eight and six) who were now with her. She had decided to have the fourth child (now four) adopted. He had always been difficult and she had never 'got on' with him. The social worker had reassured her that she had a good home for him. She was uncertain what to do about the baby. She could not cope with babies and their crying; on the other hand she feared her boyfriend would leave her if she had it adopted. Inquiries about the boyfriend revealed that he beat her but perhaps she 'deserved it'. Her husband had always been too soft and she did not fancy him sexually. She liked men to give her a good time and take her out. The doctor suggested that there seemed to be a contradiction between wanting a good time but needing to be punished for it. She laughingly agreed, then said she hated being told what to do. This was interpreted as the doctor and social worker telling her what to do (about contraception and about adoption). She then talked again about her dilemma over the new baby, about wanting him and not wanting him. Perhaps, it was suggested, this was the same as her feelings about sterilisation. She requested it, but then took her own discharge. It seemed to reflect her feelings about the baby. If she had him adopted she would want another, hence she must preserve her fertility. She looked thoughtful at this.

During the following year Mrs W.'s life renewed its chaotic pattern. She took the pill erratically, decided to be sterilised, changed her mind, finally agreed to have the fourth child adopted but decided to keep the baby. However, the latter was in and out of care much as the fourth child had been and, indeed, as the social worker had feared. The relationship with the boyfriend was unstable, which played havoc with the pill-taking. When he left she stopped taking it. When he returned she restarted. Eventually the inevitable happened and she was pregnant again. This time she decided she wanted an abortion and sterilisation. This was arranged. When seen five months later she looked well and happy. The boyfriend had finally left and she seemed pleased by this. She spoke with great warmth of the three older children who were still with her and how they took care of her. The baby was still in care but she would have him back when he was three. Her husband came to see her and the children regularly and she had no regrets about the operation.

It is difficult to be certain whether that is the end of the story.

Mrs W. may leave again if things get on top of her or she may come to regret the sterilisation and focus all her discontents on it. Having failed as a mother she might want to attempt to remedy the situation by having another child. Perhaps she will settle down to enjoy the children she has.

Although this may seem an extreme case, nevertheless many of the features shown here are typical of many cases shared between the Haringey Domiciliary Family Planning Service and Haringey Social Services:

(1) Several small children in close succession. These can overwhelm the emotional and financial resources, particularly of young, immature parents.

(2) Women who 'miss out' their teenage years by becoming pregnant and having children often need to recapture them later. This can lead to neglect of the children. The woman may have become pregnant as a teenager in an attempt to secure a stable family environment. This occurs particularly in girls from deprived backgrounds such as Mrs W.'s.

(3) A history of parental neglect is often associated with later difficulties in appreciating the continuing care that children need. It may also result in the parent looking for care from the child — 'parenting the parent', as happened with Mrs W.

(4) Impulsive immature behaviour (from whatever cause) tends to be associated with non-use or erratic use of contraception with the risk of unwanted pregnancies.

In Mrs W.'s case her unpredictable behaviour resulted from her conflict between the wish for a stable life and motherhood and the desire for a 'good time'. She had no model of a stable mother, hence her distress and anger when the first social worker left. Hurt and rejected by her mother, she nevertheless envied her apparent freedom and gaity. She loved her father but also despised him for not being able to control her mother. These feelings were later transferred to her husband. Without 'inner control' she looked to others for control, though found this difficult to accept. Her very inadequacy as a mother made her get pregnant in the hope that she could prove she was different from her mother — that she could be a good mother. However, each time she found the demands of babies and small children too great.

Sustained support over a considerable time is needed for such women until they can take responsibility for themselves with contraception. It is essential for the woman to be supported in her choice of method. This enables her to learn about her own limitations in using it. This applies particularly to the pill, cap and safe period. In Mrs W.'s case sterilisation (the 'outside' control) proved to be the only answer. However, this can only be done when the woman wants it and should never be imposed.

(5) This case illustrates the enormous demands which can be made on the social worker. It would have been easy to overlook the contraceptive issue in the midst of all the problems faced by this family. And yet further pregnancies would (and indeed did) exacerbate them. The domiciliary service was able to lift some of this burden from the social worker.

(6) Finally, this family demonstrates the tragic situation of some children born to immature parents, who become pawns and shuttlecocks, while the parents themselves are desperately trying to grow up.

13
Groups that need Special Care with Contraception

The groups that need special care with contraception are those most vulnerable to an unwanted pregnancy and/or those whose physical and emotional resources would be overwhelmed by any or further pregnancies. The social worker may well be involved with members of these groups in the community, either as separate individuals or as one of a whole family. In other instances the social worker may be providing care in a residential setting, e.g. for the handicapped or children 'in care'. By being aware of those most at risk the social worker can introduce the topic of contraception at an appropriate time. This may be in terms of *family limitation* for those who would be overwhelmed by another pregnancy, *family spacing* to provide a rest for the mother, *prevention of pregnancy* altogether, particularly for the young teenager or severely handicapped.

The positive benefits of contraception and family planning need to be stressed. Where there is ambivalence about a possible pregnancy, particularly in the case of the young teenager who 'needs a baby' as a solution to other difficulties, dealing with contraception will only be part of the care needed. In these cases work will have to be done with the whole family to explore why the teenager needs to resort to such desperate measures. The social worker will also need to decide what is the best means of providing contraceptive advice — through clinics, GP or domiciliary service. Where the latter exists it is often the most appropriate means for those whose motivation is poor and who need most support. The following groups are dealt with:

a) the young. Since contraception and the young cannot be divorced from the other issues surrounding young people and sex, these will be looked at together.

b) the single-parent family:
   i) the unmarried mother;
   ii) divorced and separated;
c) families with emotional and mental difficulties;

d) large families;
e) the handicapped.

THE YOUNG

The young person is faced with various tasks in becoming an adult. These are concerned with finding out who he is (the identity crisis), what he will be and do and establishing emotional independence from the family. In addition he has to come to terms with his own sexuality and form completely new (to him) relationships — sexual ones. The sex drive is both the spur and the means of the young person seeking relationships outside the home so that eventually he will leave the family and form one of his own.

Adolescence is a time of change both physically and emotionally. The body grows rapidly and the sexual organs mature. These changes begin around 11—13 years (puberty). Girls tend to develop earlier than boys by two years and hence may prefer the company of older boys. The average age for the first period (the menarche) is now twelve years. Seminal emission begins at about fourteen. Emotionally there are unpredictable mood swings caused by hormonal changes. The adolescent can regress to childhood dependence one minute and demand to be treated like an adult the next. While their children are bursting with energy and vigour, parents may be trying to cope with the stresses of middle age — the loss of youth and sexual attractiveness. Thus it is hardly, perhaps, surprising that there are tensions — jealousies and rivalries within the family, especially between the adolescent and the same-sex parent. To deal successfully with adolescents requires maturity and stability. Parents need to be able to affirm the sexual attractiveness of the adolescent without being seductive. This non-demanding affirmation, especially for teenage girls, prevents their needing to test it prematurely outside the family, often with disastrous results. Parents tend to view their adolescents' developing sexuality with mixed feelings — pride, envy and fear. If fear and envy predominate, the parents may deny any expression of sexuality and treat their teenage children as though they were much younger. Should they discover that their child is sexually active they react with shocked horror, exemplified by the phrase 'my little girl is not old enough for that'. Other parents anxious about normality, e.g. heterosexuality, may push their child into premature sexual experimentation. Yet others obtain vicarious pleasure from their adolescents' sexual exploits. This refers to those parents who feel they 'missed out' on their teenage years. Publicly they present themselves as liberated and understanding parents. They may also react with mock horror.

How well the adolescent copes with his sexuality and the other changes depends both on present family relationships and on early childhood experience. Where this has been an unhappy one, sex may be used to gain attention or deliberately to punish the parents and hurt others and the self. Thus boys who have a poor relationship with their mothers may deliberately exploit girls sexually and make them pregnant. Idealisation of the mother can have a similar effect in that boys will have sex only with girls they despise. Girls whose fathers behave seductively towards them may become 'boy mad' in order to escape incestuous involvement. The parental relationship itself will often determine the kind of relationships the teenager makes. For example, where parents are continually arguing and finding fault with each other, the young person is likely to develop a disillusioned and cynical view of relationships between the sexes. If the father is henpecked the son may despise him and attempt to revenge himself on women by using them sexually, though he may be secretly afraid of them.

Societal attitudes towards young people and sex

These are inconsistent and confused. There are no norms or accepted codes of sexual behaviour for young people in Western society. Many primitive societies have acknowledged adolescent sexuality and have devised ways of dealing with it (Henriques 1959). Not only is Western society confused in its attitudes towards adolescent sexuality, it also imposes enormous commercial pressures on young people. It allows the insecurity associated with adolescence to be exploited, especially in relation to sex. For example, it has been estimated that the 3 million 12—18-year-old girls in Britain today spend £57.5 million on cosmetics and toiletries. Teenagers are good for business. These pressures need to be taken into account when teenagers are criticised. The permissive society, as Meyerson (1975) has observed, is always about other people and adolescents. Thus the impression is often given by the media that all fourteen-year-old girls are on the pill or having abortions.

Sexual relationships in the young

Marriages are no longer arranged and there are no chaperones. Indeed the young person is expected to find a partner, often with little preparation. To do this they must package themselves as attractively as possible in the current sexy image. This exposes the young person to the pain and humiliation of rejection — of being found wanting or lacking in some respect. At a time when the individual should be exploring all kinds of relationships with both the same and the opposite sex, there are enormous pressures to get the whole business over with as quickly as possible by 'going steady', particularly for young working-class people. This usually means forming an intense possessive relationship. When young people do start to go out with each other, girls (but not boys) are usually warned to 'be careful' (of pregnancy). Once a relationship is started the question of 'how far to go' soon overshadows everything else. For boys anxious to prove themselves it is 'going as far as she will let you' or 'going further than you did the time before'. The sex urge is particular strong in boys at this time. (Kinsey *et al.* (1948) found the male sexual peak was around 17—18 years with frequent erections and need for ejaculation). At this age girls tend to be seen as a sexual challenge. For both sexes there is a need both to satisfy sexual curiosity and to ascertain whether they will perform adequately.

Girls tend to be expected by both parents and society to be the guardians of sexual morality — to control how far the boy goes. Hence their indignation — 'boys are only after one thing' — to which boys respond, 'If she wasn't asking for it she shouldn't have dressed that way'. Another frequent comment heard from boys is that if they do not make a sexual advance early on in the relationship the girl will think they are a 'poof' or queer. These comments reflect the long-held views of sexual roles — the female has to attract and wait for the male to pursue and risk rejection. Both sexes may be trapped by their role expectation and fail to appreciate the other's position. Thus it is as hurtful for the girl not to be pursued as it is for the boy to be rejected.

Further pressures to be coped with are those exerted by the peer group — the teasing and boasting about sexual exploits. Information about sex is mainly gained from friends (Schofield 1965, Farrell 1978). Belief that one's friends are all having sex may force some young people into having sex prematurely.

Young people also have fears about 'normality' and proof of this is sought by having intercourse. Girls doubtful of their attractiveness may see the promise of sex as the only thing they can offer. For those young people who find it difficult to relate to others, sex may be all that is shared. For yet others with limited abilities and poor future prospects, sex may provide the only excitement in otherwise dull lives.

Pressures by boys on girls to have sex can vary from the crude 'You're frigid' to the subtle 'You don't really love me'. It takes enormous self-confidence to refuse sex when these pressures are sustained. Should intercourse be allowed to happen it is usually sanctioned by 'being in love' − romantic love, a somewhat ethereal state, 'natural' and spontaneous, which tends to preclude the use of contraception. Romantic love is also the basis of marriage and 'living happily ever after'. (What is rarely made clear to young people is that romantic love consists largely of sexual attraction which may be temporary and that loving someone, working at love, is vastly different from being in love (Fromm 1965, Rollo May, 1969)).

Thus there may be a denial that sexual intercourse is taking place until a crisis such as a venereal infection or a pregnancy occurs. The girl who becomes pregnant may protest that sex only happened once or that a boy took advantage of her or that it happened when she got drunk at a party.

When pregnancy does occur it precipitates a crisis in the relationship usually before the young couple have learnt very much about themselves or each other. This imposes strains that the relationship cannot withstand. The couple are forced to make a decision for which they are ill-prepared. Hence bewilderment ('Why did it have to happen?') and resentment ('It's your fault') come between the boy and girl. He feels trapped. He was only having sex − it wasn't serious. She feels hurt and rejected. She loved him and look what has happened. Sometimes the girl has fantasies when initially hearing that she is pregnant that all will be well − he will be delighted, they will marry and live happily ever after. The shock when he does not respond in this way may leave a bitter scar. 'Boys are no good, they're only after one thing.' Abortion may be seen as the quick and easy solution. However, unless counselling and support is offered at this time, the guilt associated with the abortion may result in the girl getting pregnant soon afterwards to make amends. Adoption is also a painful solution. Keeping the baby may seem the most acceptable solution. Unfortunately, the baby may be rejected and even if it is not the difficulties and hardship facing the unmarried mother are enormous. If the couple decide to marry 'for the sake of the baby' there may be increasing resentment that turns into hostility and even violence and the baby may be a pawn between the couple. What is the solution? Some would argue that no sex before marriage is the answer, others that all girls should be put on the pill at the age of puberty. Neither approach is appropriate or helpful. What is far more important and relevant is to accept that adolescents are sexual people and that though they may not be actually having intercourse (nor want to for some time) the possibility that they will exists. This acceptance by both parents and professional workers means that the dialogue about sex with young people can begin on a realistic basis with preparation for a sexual relationship. Within this context discussion about caring about other people and not using them for one's own gratification can take place (of course, if this kind of caring is not shown within the family, such discussion may well seem hypocritical to the young person). Information about contraception and sexually transmitted disease should also be given, and about where to obtain advice. Caring for someone includes using contraception and preventing the transmission of infection. Contrary to expectation, such discussion is more likely to make the young person stop and think before embarking on a sexual relationship rather than rushing into one.

Facts about teenagers

As mentioned earlier, the media often convey the impression that all young people are sexually active. How true is this? Two British studies (Schofield 1965, Farrell 1978) carried out ten years apart showed that, although the proportion of young people admitting to sexual experience has risen, it is still a minority. Thus in Schofield's sample of 1,800 young people, 20% of boys and 12% of girls had had intercourse by the age of 19; 6 per cent of fifteen-year-old boys and 2 per cent of fifteen-year-old girls interviewed were sexually experienced. Farrell found that twenty-six per cent of boys and twelve per cent of girls claimed to have had their first sexual experience before the age of sixteen. However, less than half (48 per cent) of the single teenagers had had intercourse by the age of nineteen. From the evidence Farrell concluded that 1 girl in 8 was likely to have intercourse before the age of sixteen.

In both studies class differences were shown. Thus working-class young people (particularly boys) were more likely than middle-class young people to be sexually experienced earlier.

Unfortunately, since young people (like their elders) are not always very responsible about their sexual behaviour, there have been casualties. There has been a rise both in the number of pregnancies in the under-twenties and in the incidence of sexually transmitted disease.

Illegitimate births to teenagers

In 1976, 37 per cent of all illegitimate births were to girls under twenty, compared to 15 per cent in 1951. Among the under-sixteen's the number increased from 200 in 1951 to 1,414 in 1976. Fortunately the number of illegitimate births per 1,000 girls in any age group has begun to drop since the 1970s. In 1975 half the babies born to married teenagers were conceived before marriage; 1 in 250 girls reaching their sixteenth birthday and 1 in 125 girls reaching their seventeenth birthday will now have an illegitimate baby (Social Trends 1978).

Table 1: Illegitimate live births to teenagers

England & Wales	Scotland

Girls 16—19 years

England & Wales	Scotland
1970 = 19,460	1971 = 2,144
1971 = 20,042	1972 = 2,215
1972 = 20,150	1973 = 2,224
1973 = 19,045	1974 = 2,313
1974 = 19,308	
1975 = 19,001	
1976 = 18,405	
1977 = 18,761	

Girls under 16 years

1951 =	200
1970 =	1,403
1971 =	1,513
1972 =	1,587
1973 =	1,678
1974 =	1,553
1975 =	1,489
1976 =	1,414
1977 =	1,281

Source: *OPCS*

Abortion and the teenager

In 1969, 18 per cent (10,166) of all abortions performed in England and Wales were carried out on girls under twenty. By 1977 the proportion had risen to 27 per cent (28,215). Among the under-sixteens abortions rose from 1,732 in 1970 to 3,624 in 1977. The numbers appear to be stabilising since 1975 among older teenagers. This is thought to be due to improved contraceptive practice consequent upon society's changing attitudes towards young people and sex rather than to a decrease in sexual activity. This view is shared by several authors (Thompson 1976, Edmunds & Yarrow 1977, Bone 1978). Unfortunately, however, the number of abortions appears to be increasing among younger teenagers. The under-sixteens also tend to seek abortion later than other groups. 28 per cent of all abortions on girls under sixteen were carried out at over thirteen weeks pregnancy compared to 18 per cent for the 25–29 age group (Abortion Statistics 1975).

Table 2 : Abortion to girls under 20

England & Wales	Scotland	England & Wales under 16
1971 = 25,611	1971 = 1,234	2,296
1972 = 31,281	1972 = 1,685	2,804
1973 = 31,838	1973 = 1,853	3,090
1974 = 27,005	1974 = 1,969	3,335
1975 = 27,395		3,570
1976 = 27,388		3,425
1977 = 28,215 (27 per cent of total number of abortions)		3,624

(Source: OPCS Ref. AB 78/5 AB 78/10)

Sexually transmitted diseases

The incidence of gonorrhoea (the most prevalent venereal disease) has risen dramatically in the under-twenties, so that one in five of all cases occur in a person under the age of twenty. This is dealt with more fully in Part 4.

Young people most at risk from pregnancy

Teenagers who become pregnant are considered in Part 3. Since pregnancy in the teenager often has disastrous consequences for the girl herself, her family and the baby (where she chooses to go through with the pregnancy), every attempt should be made to prevent such a situation occurring. It is proposed here to look at those teenagers who are most at risk of becoming pregnant. By being aware of them the social worker may be able to take preventive action. The social worker may already be involved with such teenagers — through the school, at a child guidance clinic or in a residential home, or indirectly through involvement with the whole family. The social worker may be forced to make a choice that is at variance with parental wishes about contraceptive advice for the teenager at risk. Obviously, each case must be treated with great care. Those teenagers who start to have sex in their early teens are at great risk. A separate group of teenagers may deliberately seek to become pregnant and want a baby very much, though for the wrong reasons.

Characteristics of girls at risk from pregnancy

1. Lack of self-esteem and poor self-image

The girl who lacks self-esteem and who has not done well at school or whose parents are over-ambitious for her may get involved in a sexual relationship where pregnancy is allowed to happen. For those girls who do not know what to do with their lives, motherhood may be seen as a solution. Motherhood can also solve the identity crisis and answer the question 'Who am I?' Lack of self-esteem is often caused by or associated with uncertainty about sexuality and fertility. The girl who fears she may be sterile owing to mistaken ideas about, for example, excess body hair, small breasts or scanty periods may seek to become pregnant as a reassurance of femininity and fertility. The girl who lacks self-esteem is often strongly influenced by friends and the peer group. She may feel that the only way to prove to them that she really is sexually desirable is to become pregnant. The girl who has no belief in herself may not believe that her boyfriend can really love her; again proof may be sought by becoming pregnant. Where sex itself is felt to be bad the girl may get pregnant to make it good.

The school social worker may be asked to see the girl because she appears isolated and withdrawn or easily led and getting into trouble or because she is working badly or is absent repeatedly from school. She may be behaving in a sexually provocative way. The girl herself may seek help because she is depressed or fears she is pregnant.

2. Girls from unhappy or unstable backgrounds

The girl who feels unloved and rejected or is compared unfavourably to siblings may look for love outside the home. She soon discovers that sex is a way of obtaining attention. The risk of pregnancy is then high, as no thought is given to contraception. For some girls there is a desperate need for parental substitutes. Failure to find these within the family may lead the girl to place a boyfriend in this role. The girl's expectations of him are usually too great and she then focuses her needs on the desire for a baby. This can become an obsession where the reality of caring for a child plays little or no part. The baby is seen as someone who will give her the love denied by parents and boyfriend. Unfortunately for the girl, the baby's needs are as great as her own.

Anger with the parents and their treatment of her may make the girl deliberately seek pregnancy to punish them and to demonstrate that she can be a better parent (Spicer 1975). A girl with over-protective and controlling parents or with parents who exploit her to care for them and the family may see a baby as the only means of establishing her independence and rights as a separate person. (This occurs particularly with girls of West Indian origin.)

Parental marital conflict can cause the teenage girl to seek affection elsewhere. Again pregnancy may be seen as a means of escape from the burden of pain and misery and the conflict of loyalties engendered. Sometimes these girls can deceive the worker by hiding their distress by a blasé, off-hand manner as if the parents' problems had nothing whatever to do with her. This pain must be reached for the girl to be helped. Another response by the girl to parental conflict and one which is easy to ignore, certainly, within a school context, is withdrawal. Again such a girl is at risk from pregnancy. When pregnancy does happen it often occasions surprise, since the girl is 'no trouble to anyone'. Discovery of parental infidelity, particularly that of the father, by the teenage girl can have serious consequences. The girl may become promiscuous as if to demonstrate that sex means nothing. By going from man to man she proves to herself that men are really no good and only want sex. Again pregnancy is a risk because the girl in her defiance is unlikely to be responsible about contraception.

Thus the teenage girl who is under stress from whatever cause may be at risk from pregnancy. Initially she may flaunt her sexuality as a means of getting attention and if this fails become pregnant. The teenage girl in this situation is often scapegoated as 'the problem' and presented for help as being beyond control. In extreme cases the parents may even attempt to pressurise the social worker to take the girl into care. It is usually the parents' marriage which is at fault and in need of help as well as the girl herself. Thus work with the whole family and the parents' marriage in particular may be necessary.

Although the position of the girl has been stressed, almost as though she became pregnant in isolation, much of what has been said also relates to boys. Lack of belief in themselves and/or concern about virility may cause them to get a girl pregnant. The ability to do so may be a compensation for failure in other areas of their lives.

Two other groups of young people at risk from pregnancy are:

3. Those in care

These girls are one of the most vulnerable groups of young people, not only because they usually come from disturbed backgrounds but also because of the added strain of being in care — separated from brothers and sisters, rarely visited by their families and having no one to call their own. Their feelings of rejection can be overwhelming and they find it difficult to trust anyone. As a result they are at particular risk of becoming pregnant in their early teens. Sometimes with the impending end of the care order the girl, fearful of independence, may become pregnant so that she can go on being cared for. (14 per cent of the 400 unmarried mothers [this figure includes girls of West Indian origin] referred for domiciliary family planning care in Haringey between 1968 and 1976 had been in care for a substantial part of their childhood. The majority (88 per cent) got pregnant between the ages of 13 and 16.)

Illustrative case: Phyllis was sixteen years old, overweight though pretty. She never knew her parents, having been put into care at the age of two. She lived in a fantasy dream world.

Her men friends all loved her passionately and could not live without her but in reality they never stayed very long. She became pregnant. She loved the baby intensely though she neglected him and he had to be taken in care for a short time. The baby's father left her for another girl. She then had a succession of boyfriends and contracted VD. She was referred for domiciliary family planning after the birth of the baby. She refused advice because 'there was no point', she 'wasn't doing nothing'. The domiciliary doctor kept in touch, visiting regularly every 6—8 weeks trying to build up a relationship. Phyllis manipulated relationships, played off one worker against another and told lies. She found it very hard to trust anyone or to believe that anyone could really care, which was hardly surprising given the fact that she had been in six different homes while in care. Eventually she decided to take the pill. She required intensive visiting, and even so her pill-taking was erratic. She became pregnant and had an abortion (because the boy left her on learning that she was pregnant) and was fitted with a coil. She kept this for two years. She then met a married man whose wife was unable to have children. She fantasised that if she had a baby he would leave his wife for her. She had the coil removed and became pregnant. The man kept promising to leave his wife but never did. Phyllis is now left with two children by two different fathers. Without the support of the domiciliary service it is unlikely that she would have persevered as she did with contraception. Thus at least she has a three-year gap between the first child and the second. This is vital since her emotional resources and patience are so limited that if she had had several children close together it is likely that one or more would have been taken into care. She has been refitted with a coil and is ever hopeful of meeting 'Mr Right' who will take care of her. The domiciliary service still visits.

The tragedy for girls in both groups (2) and (3) is that they often have strong fantasies of a happy but idealised family life. Since they feel powerless to do anything about their family of origin, they feel that the solution lies in the creation of their own family. Their immaturity makes this extremely difficult. The boys they go out with may not be looking for love but for sex. They are not usually thinking of settling down at this age. The girl, though, is looking for love. Contraception may well not be used or even thought of in these circumstances. It is unlikely that she will go to the clinic on her own. Should the girl become pregnant she may well not want an abortion, since a baby is what she really wants.

These are often very difficult and time-consuming cases since these girls need so much support, both emotional and physical. Prevention of this situation obviously lies not just in the provision of contraception but in a continuing caring one-to-one relationship to help the girl value herself. Other ways of helping may be to involve the girl in the care of babies and small children, or in group work with other girls in a similar situation.

4. *Teenage girls of West Indian origin*

The cultural situation has a strong influence on young West Indian teenagers to get pregnant, though there are other pressures. These will be looked at more fully in Chapter 14. Again the provision of contraception is not enough, though it may need to be part of the help given.

West Indian girls who are in care often become so at the time of adolescence as being beyond parental control. This usually refers to staying out late and going out with boys. There is parental fear of pregnancy in this situation.

Young people's clinics

Much anxiety has been expressed about Young People's Clinics, which offer contraceptive advice to the single. They are believed by some people to encourage promiscuity and it is said that if they did not exist then young people would not have sex. The evidence at present available from studies of the clientele of such clinics shows that the majority of girls attending have already embarked on a sexual relationship — very few are virgins.

What kind of girl does attend the clinic? After ten years' experience at such a clinic in North London, I have found that she is usually about 17—18 years old; having had one or two short-lived sexual relationships she is now going steady, though may not see herself actually marrying the present boyfriend. The couple have usually relied on a mixture of withdrawal, safe period and sheath. A possible pregnancy scare and/or the relationship becoming more serious has led the girl to come to the clinic. She has usually heard about the clinic from a friend. She is usually middle-class, has a firm sense of her own identity and accepts her sexuality as a good part of herself. Her parents have usually been able to discuss sex openly with her and, though not necessarily approving of premarital sex, have indicated that should she become sexually involved then it would be preferable for her to use an effective form of birth control. Thus she is able to make a conscious decision about contraception. It takes courage to go to a clinic or doctor since society does not make it easy to make such a rational decision. Such girls may go steady for several months or years and may eventually marry the boy. They may live with their partners before marriage. Should the relationship end it is not an infrequent occurrence for the girl to attend the clinic and say that she no longer wants the pill (the pill being the most popular method chosen) but will return when she does. Or she may continue with the pill as it makes her periods lighter and prevents menstrual pains, even though she is not having intercourse.

Another kind of girl commonly seen at the clinic is from a working-class background and has had the same boyfriend from her early teens. A point is reached in the relationship where sex can be allowed, as there is a definite commitment on his part to marriage some time in the future.

The working-class girl suffers more from the double standard of morality than the middle-class girl. In the past she may have used her sexuality or the promise of sex as a bait to get a husband (beautifully portrayed by Stan Barstow's novel, *A Kind of Loving*). With the fear of pregnancy removed by the advent of the pill, pressure is put on her to have intercourse. For such a girl, going to the clinic for the pill before intercourse poses all kinds of dilemma. 'If I go on the pill all the boys will think I'm available.' Deep down she may fear that she will become promiscuous. Thus as she is 'not that kind of girl', a bad sexy girl, she may not go to the clinic until she has a pregnancy scare. Her ambivalence may show up at the initial interview with statements such as 'The pill is unnatural. It's not really safe. I shall get fat.' Implicit in all this is, 'I really shouldn't take it because I don't really want to have sex.' But she may fear losing her boyfriend. A quiet seventeen-year-old who had been attending the clinic for about six months suddenly lashed out one evening, 'If it wasn't for the pill I wouldn't be having sex.' She liked her boyfriend but did not want sex because she did not want to let her parents down. She told him she was afraid of getting pregnant but he persistently badgered her to take the pill and so she came to the clinic. She had been unable to voice her resentment initially but the deceit involved in carrying on the sexual relationship, always fearing to be found out, was too much for her. The relationship ended soon after.

The under-sixteens

One of the most difficult issues concerning young people is the appropriate age of consent. At present it is sixteen years for girls. There is no age of consent for boys apart from that concerned with homosexual relationships, which is twenty-one. Physical maturity is occurring earlier (one eleven-year-old and three twelve year-olds had live births in 1976). Emotional maturity does not have such a clear demarcation. The controversy about the age of consent is about emotional maturity and readiness for a sexual relationship and the possible harmful effects it may have on the girl and her ability to make mature relationships in the future. There is little statistical evidence about this. Some doctors working in young people's clinics have advocated that the age of consent be lowered. One doctor (Hutchinson 1976) noted that many sixteen-year-olds who arrived at her clinic soon after their sixteenth birthdays had been having regular intercourse for some months prior to that. She felt that by keeping the age of consent at sixteen these girls were prevented from seeking help and were running the risk of unwanted pregnancy. It is a difficult and contradictory situation. On the one hand there is a law which makes it an absolute offence for a man to have intercourse with a girl under thirteen and an offence for a man to have intercourse with a girl between thirteen and sixteen unless the man believes himself to be married to the girl or being under twenty-four, he believes her to be over sixteen, and on the other hand there is the advice from the DHSS to doctors that it is for the doctor to decide whether to provide contraceptive advice and treatment for a girl under sixteen. If he acted in good faith in protecting the girl against the potentially harmful effects of intercourse, he would not be charged with aiding and abetting. He is advised to seek the girl's consent to tell her parents, but failure to do so would not put the doctor in jeopardy. The under-sixteens form about 3—5 per cent of the clientele of Brook Young Peoples' Clinics (Brook 1978). About 3 per cent of the girls (108 out of a total of 3,600) attending the YPC in Haringey between 1968 and 1976 were under sixteen. Two-thirds were brought or referred by social workers and were either under a supervision order or in care of the local authority. About a third were pregnant, and half of these pregnancies were terminated while half the girls carried on with the pregnancy and had the baby.

The difficulties facing parents when their young teenage daughter gets involved in a sexual relationship and who love and care about their children is illustrated by the following case. A fifteen-year-old girl, Christine, attended an ordinary birth control session. The doctor at the clinic was not happy to see someone under the age of consent and referred her to the YPC. Christine had been having intercourse for three months but the boyfriend disliked the sheath, which he had used occasionally. His mother knew they were having sex and told them to go to a clinic. Christine wanted the pill. The doctor felt they were behaving responsibly and prescribed it. A week later, Christine's mother phoned the doctor and demanded to know why Christine was on the pill. (She had found a packet in a drawer.) The doctor suggested they all get together to discuss the situation. The parents were concerned for their daughter. They liked the boy and did not want to break up the relationship, but they wanted Christine to stop having intercourse. After much discussion and weeping by mother and Christine, Christine promised not to have sex. She kept her promise for four months. They then had intercourse, the sheath slipped off and pregnancy resulted. Termination was requested and arranged, and at a subsequent discussion the parents decided to let Christine take the pill. They were not happy about it but realised that short of locking Christine up or forcing her to leave the boy (which might have resulted in Christine leaving home — she was approaching sixteen) there was not much else they could do. They also wanted her to go to college to be a hairdresser, which she had always wanted to do. Christine is now nineteen years old, still at home, and gets on well with her parents. She attends college and still has the same boyfriend.

Promiscuity

It was noted earlier that there was concern lest YPCs should encourage promiscuity. Promiscuity is an emotive word and means different things to different people depending on the society and mores of that society. For example, among many Mediterranean people where virginity is considered vital for any girl who wants to marry, any sexual involvement before marriage will be considered promiscuous. In Western society it can mean having three or four sexual partners before marriage, or the bed-hopping fantasy of popular imagination. Promiscuity is defined in the *Shorter Oxford English Dictionary* as 'casual, carelessly irregular sexual relationships'. There is no evidence, despite public fears, that young people are promiscuous (Schofield 1965, Farrell 1978).

At the young people's clinic in Haringey, apart from discussion about the risks of venereal disease, no attempt is made to pry into the sexual behaviour of the people attending. Over the years it has been possible to gather information about it in an unobtrusive way. Some girls have only one sexual partner and marry him. Others have 2−3 brief affairs and then a long-lasting relationship which leads to marriage. A third pattern may be described as serial monogamy, each relationship lasting several months or years with gaps in between. The general impression of girls attending is that the young are more accepting of sex as a natural enjoyable function. Given the past inhibited behaviour and confused fearful attitudes towards sex, it is perhaps not surprising that the old should envy the young.

THE ONE-PARENT FAMILY

The number of one-parent families has been increasing steadily. Figures released by the OPCS in 1978 showed that the number had risen to 750,000 as compared with 570,000 in 1971. This is mainly attributed to an increase in the number of broken marriages. General Household Survey data suggest that by 1976 one-parent families had come to constitute 11 per cent of all families with dependent children (compared with 8 per cent in 1971), three-quarters of them living with no other adult person in the household.

The one-parent family (single, divorced, separated, widowed) is under tremendous financial and emotional stress. The majority are mothers alone with children. The poverty and loneliness experienced by so many of these women make them vulnerable to exploitation by men seeking sexual relationships without commitment. Mothers alone with children have attested to this in sociological studies (Gill 1977). This illustrates the survival of the double standard of morality. The social worker is likely to have a number of such women on his case-load and should be aware of their special vulnerability. Such women may see no point in using contraception since they may not be having sex on a regular basis. Nevertheless there is a risk of unintended pregnancies.

The unmarried mother

10 per cent of the children in single-parent families belong to young unmarried mothers. Attitudes towards illegitimacy have tended to be (and still are to a certain extent) punitive. This occasionally took extreme forms in the past. Instances are known of unmarried mothers being institutionalised in mental homes for no other reason than that they were unmarried mothers. Unmarried fathers have never come in for such condemnation. In Victorian times unmarried mothers were often forced to abandon or kill their infants since their future prospects with them were so bleak.

Since illegitimacy is deviant in the sense that most children are born in wedlock, various attempts to explain why some women become unmarried mothers have been made over the years. Vincent (1966) has shown that studies made in the 1920s stressed 'immorality' and 'mental deficiency'. During the 1930s findings emphasised the importance of 'broken homes' and 'poverty'. In the 1940s and 1950s psychological processes were stressed, such as 'unresolved parent child' conflicts. As mentioned earlier, fertility studies have ignored out-of-wedlock pregnancies since they represent a small proportion of all births. Information about unmarried mothers tends to come from small samples. These may well be biased as they are taken from special settings such as social agencies and charity institutions.

During the 1960s both the absolute number of illegitimate births and the illegitimacy rates (i.e. ratio of illegitimate births to legitimate births) rose dramatically, especially among the under-twenties (Pearce & Farid 1977). In 1967, 1 in 12 babies born in Britain was illegitimate compared to 1 in 21 in 1957. What had brought this about? Explanations based on widespread mental illness or moral degeneracy were hardly tenable. Much more pertinent was the altered social climate, together with a change in sexual norms and the altered status of women. This has been extensively explored by Gill (1977). In the 1960s there was in increase in economic prosperity and increased mobility. The young in particular enjoyed greater freedom together with greater economic power. Sexual codes were less strict. Premarital sex, though not necessarily condoned, was more tolerated, especially for engaged couples or couples in a steady relationship. Illegitimacy itself began to carry less social stigma and girls felt less obliged to marry the father. It was increasingly recognised that 'shot-gun' marriages for the sake of the baby were only a temporary solution and might well end in divorce. Thus there was less pressure from parents and welfare agencies for the girl to marry. These changes have persisted into the 1970s, but with the advent of the Abortion Act of 1967 there has been a decrease in the absolute number of illegitimate births, though the rates have remained the same: 1 in 11 in 1975. There has also been a greater tendency for girls to keep their babies. The number of illegitimate babies adopted in 1961 was about 10,000 (62 per cent of all adoptions). By 1976 this figure had dropped to 5,000 (27 per cent of all adoptions).

The illegitimacy rate is different for the varied ethnic groups. In several London boroughs the percentage of illegitimate births is of the order of 16 per cent (that is, 1 baby in 6 is illegitimate). This is probably due to the presence of a large West Indian population. However, in cultures where illegitimacy carries a social stigma and may hinder marriage prospects (such as the Asian and Cypriot) for the girl who becomes pregnant outside marriage only three alternatives are available, to have an abortion, to have the child adopted or to marry the father. (Among unmarried mothers, excluding those of West Indian origin, referred for domiciliary family planning advice in Haringey during 1968—76 there were 2 Cypriot, 3 Asian and 12 Irish. 119 were English/Scots/Welsh. One Cypriot mother married, the other had her child adopted, as did the three Asian women. Of the 132 other unmarried mothers, only 2 had their babies adopted.

Illegitimacy — an historical perspective

Is legitimacy the norm in most societies? The concept of a principle of legitimacy has been put forward which is cross-cultural and obtains in primitive pre-literate as well as literate societies (Malinowski 1930). Only in the West Indies and American Negro society as the result of their unique and terrible history, has illegitimacy become the norm, so that no stigma is attached to it or felt by those who are illegitimate. (Illegitimacy rates are as high as 70 per cent on some West Indian islands.)

That illegitimate births have always occurred is evident from historical studies. Laslett (1976) has shown by means of parish registers that illegitimate births have always occurred, but the ratios have varied. They were low until the late sixteenth century, when they rose to 4.5 per cent. They fell during the seventeenth century possibly as a result of Puritan influence and rose again in the eighteenth century. Illegitimacy in pre-industrial England and Scotland was higher in rural than town areas and higher in the west and north-west. It also tended to run in families (Laslett 1976). The nineteenth century saw a further increase — one birth in thirteen was illegitimate in the 1860s. An increase in illegitimate births, paradoxically, does not correspond to times of food scarcity or demographic crisis but to times of affluence. The rise of the illegitimacy rates seen in the eighteenth century owed much to the rise of capitalism (Shorter 1976). This encouraged individual enterprise and self-interest at the expense of community and family interest. Whereas previously parents had control over their children and arranged their marriages, the young themselves wanted to be free. They became concerned about their own personal happiness and wanted to choose their own partners. This in turn led to an increase in premarital sexual activity with its inevitable consequences. There also seems to be a correlation between illegitimacy and early marriage. Where late marriage is the norm, the number of illegitimate births is low. The sanctions used to ensure late marriage seem also to prevent premarital sex. (This seems to be happening in China at the present time.) The age of the mother at the birth of her first illegitimate child seems to have remained roughly the same: the late twenties for the whole period 1540—1839 (Laslett 1973). This is possibly accounted for in part by the late onset of menstruation and a high incidence of infertility due to poor diet and health. It is only in the 1960s and 1970s that the phenomenon of teenage pregnancy has been seen on such a widespread scale in Western countries.

Various studies have shown that unmarried mothers and their children are amongst the most deprived members in our society (Wimperis 1960, Wynn 1964, Marsden 1969, Finer Report 1974, Hopkinson 1976 and the Court Report 1976). Having an illegitimate baby entails a 'complex network of disadvantages'. The majority are young when pregnancy occurs, receive late and insufficient ante-natal care, and have a higher rate of still-births, premature births and low birth weight babies with all the physical disadvantages these imply (Court Report 1976). Women who bear an illegitimate child (whether married, single, divorced, separated or widowed) are predominantly from lower socio-economic groups (Gill 1977).

Although it is not known for certain how many of th‹ 100,000 children in care are illegitimate, various estimates hav‹ been given. Wimperis (1960) showed that 33 per cent o‹ children. in care in twenty-one countries and boroughs i‹ England and Wales were illegitimate; The PEP Study (Lain‹ 1972) quoted a figure of 28 per cent of all children in care Work by the NSPCC Battered Child Research Team suggests ‹ link between the refusal to give an abortion and non-accidenta‹ injury to the child by young single mothers (Violence t‹ Children 1977).

Table 3: Illegitimate Births 1954—1976

England and Wales   To the nearest 100

		Illegitimate Total No.	Ratio	%	Total No. Births
	1954	32,000	1.21	4.8	674,000
	1955	31,000	1.21	4.8	668,000
	1956	33,500	1.21	4.8	700,000
	1957	34,600	1.21	4.8	723,000
	1958	36,200	1.21	5	741,000
	1959	38,200	1.20	5	749,000
	(1960	42,700	1.18	5.5	785,000
	(1961	48,500	1.17	6	811,000
	(1962	55,400	1.15	7	839,000
Swinging	(1963	59,100	1.14	7	854,000
Sixties	(1964	63,300	1.14	7	876,000
	(1965	66,200	1.13	8	863,000
	(1966	67,000			
	1967	70,000	1.12	8	832,000
Abortion Act	1968	70,000	1.12	8	819,000
	1970	64,700	1.12	8	784,500
	1971	65,400	1.12	8	783,200
	1972	62,500	1.12	8	725,400
	1973	58,100	1.12	8	676,000
	1974	56,500	1.12	8	639,900
	1975	54,900	1.11	9	603,400
	1976	53,800	1.11	9	584,300
	1977	55,400	1.10	10	569,300
	1978*	60,600	1.10	10	596,200

*Provisional

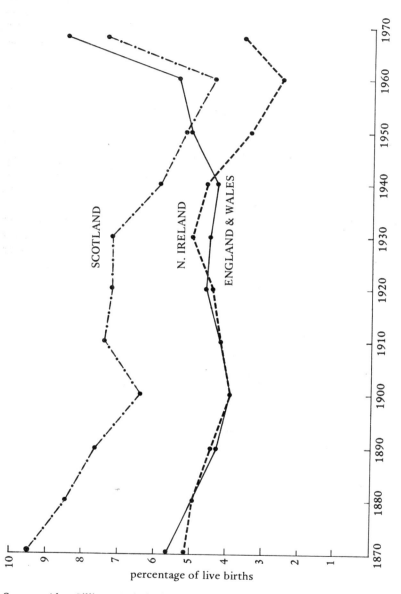

SCOTLAND

N. IRELAND

ENGLAND & WALES

percentage of live births

Source: Alan Sillitoe: *Britain in Figures; A Handbook of Social Statistics* (Pelican 1971) p.23. 'Reprinted by permission of Penguin Books Ltd.'

Teenage unmarried mothers

One in four 16—20-year-olds and two in five under-sixteens who are pregnant choose to have an illegitimate baby (Thompson 1976). Not only are these mothers more likely to suffer economic hardship, but their immaturity may make the demands of motherhood too onerous, especially where they are not supported by their family or boyfriend.

When teenage unmarried mothers are asked why they did not seek advice or use contraception, the response is often 'But I'm not that sort of girl!' That sort of girl is the girl who makes a conscious decision about her sexuality and gets contraceptive advice. For some teenage mothers a conscious decision about sex is often equated with immorality. Thus sex occurring spontaneously — 'I didn't mean it to happen' — is less immoral and can be more easily forgiven by society and the girl herself. This is somewhat analogous to the situation of premeditated murder (more wicked) versus unpremeditated murder done in a fit of passion (wicked but understandable and therefore forgivable). Thus the girl who gets pregnant in this manner may deny that she is really having sex when the pregnancy is discovered. One girl, when asked by a counsellor about the circumstances which led to the pregnancy, replied, 'And I wasn't really there!' Of course these comments are *post hoc* rationalisations of behaviour for which the girl feels guilty. And in fairness to young people, the person who gets contraceptive advice is not praised. Pregnancies in the young may occur as 'biological accidents' in that some are probably more fertile than others. Thus the story of intercourse taking place only once may be true in some cases.

There seem to be certain personality and family factors (looked at earlier) at work in some cases, particularly in young unmarried mothers and in those who, having a choice, opt to continue with pregnancy. Thus for some unmarried mothers there would seem to be a 'need for a baby'.

The pregnancy may be used to test or strengthen a relationship. Some girls have a fantasy about this: they dream of their boyfriends being delighted when they learn of the pregnancy and offering to marry them. The dream is all too often shattered by the boyfriend saying that if she sues him for maintenance, he will say all his friends had a 'poke'. Experience from an unmarried mothers' home reveals a depressingly similar reaction as related by the girls themselves: 'He didn't want to know', 'Said it must be someone else's', 'Since I let him have it [sex] I must have let someone else have it too'. These reactions reveal the shock and panic felt by the boys and the need to escape responsibility for the pregnancy. For some unmarried fathers sex is seen solely for pleasure and the connection between intercourse and procreation denied (Spicer 1975).

In some cases the boy is proud to have proof of his fertility (wrongly equated with virility), though not prepared to take care of the girl or the child.

Although the unmarried father is often considered the villain of the piece he may in fact have been used by the girl to get a baby for her own needs. This is suggested by incidents where the girl either deliberately does not tell the boy that she is pregnant or breaks off the relationship when she learns that she is pregnant. This was noted over thirty years ago by Young (1945): 'Some girls reduce the man to the position of a tool, a kind of biological accessory without reality or meaning as a person'.

Out of 136 unmarried mothers (all ages, but excluding West Indian mothers) referred to the Haringey Domiciliary Service between 1968 and 1976 (which of course is not a random sample), 60 per cent had had the experience of an unstable background (parents separated/divorced, in care during childhood or illegitimate themselves. 38 per cent came from families who were classed as multi-problem involved with the social services. Of these 136 unmarried mothers, 95 per cent had used no birth control prior to the first conception, and 68 per cent had used no birth control prior to referral to the domiciliary service. 73 per cent (100 cases) were teenagers and three-quarters of these had had their first conception at seventeen or earlier. Only 29 per cent were cohabiting with the baby's father and thirty-nine had more than one child, usually by different fathers.

A study based on interviews with 116 unmarried mothers conducted through four maternity hospitals in Edinburgh (Hopkinson 1976) revealed that 50 per cent were aged between 16 and 19 and that 81 per cent of their fathers were in social classes III, IV and V. 77 per cent of these single mothers had never used contraception and 67 per cent stated that they had received no sex education at school. One difficulty surrounding the whole question of sex education in school is how far young people see it as relevant to their needs at the time. If a girl has a need to get pregnant to give her something to love she may deny that she received any sex education in order to justify her action. 44 per cent of Hopkinson's sample came from families of five or more children. Of the 136 unmarried mothers seen by the Haringey service, 55 per cent came from families where there were five or more children. While this does not necessarily mean that unmarried mothers are more likely to come from large families, it does mean that as the mothers of these families have failed to use contraceptives themselves 'their attitudes to contraception are inevitably absorbed by their children' (Hopkinson 1976). In some large families in Haringey, once the mother has reached the menopause the single daughters may start to have children to give to the mother.

The foregoing comments about unmarried mothers are not to suggest that they are all inadequate or unable to cope. However, those from unstable or unhappy backgrounds and those who are rejected by their families will often be involved with the social services. The fragility of their relationships and their low self-esteem make them vulnerable to unintended pregnancies, and thus contraceptive help is needed.

Contraceptive help

The view has been expressed that the post-natal period should be avoided by health visitors offering contraceptive advice to single mothers (Hopkinson 1976). And indeed, during the first few months after the birth remarks such as 'I've gone off men', 'I've learnt my lesson', 'Men only want one thing' may seem to reinforce the view. However, so much depends on the way in which contraception is introduced and discussed. The time after the birth but before a new relationship is embarked upon allows experimentation with methods. Also, encouragement and support will be needed to persevere as sex may not be on a regular basis. The already low opinion that she has of herself may not only prevent her seeking contraceptive advice (since this would only confirm the opinion others have of her that she 'is no better than the should be') but also involve her in relationships with men who do 'use' her sexually. And thus she is at special risk of becoming pregnant again.

Illustrative case Shirley was sixteen years old, from a working-class background. Her father left her mother when Shirley was eleven. She had two older sisters and a younger brother. The brother was under the care of Child Guidance as he was absent frequently from school. Shirley began to go out with boys at fourteen and eventually had a steady relationship with a boy, John, four years older than herself. She did not get on with her mother and resented her telling her what to do. The relationship between them deteriorated further when Shirley began to go steady with John. Mother seemed to be jealous of their relationship. Shirley and John began to have sex but did not take precautions. When Shirley found she was pregnant she was delighted and saw the baby as a chance to escape from home. John said he would stick by her and when they had saved some money they would get married. Their relationship during the pregnancy was stormy. Shirley often felt too tired to go out and John would get bored and go off on his own. When the baby, a boy, was born they became reconciled. However, this was only temporary and the quarrelling resumed as John was jealous of the baby and resentful of the attention Shirley gave him. After the birth Shirley had been referred by the hospital social worker to the domiciliary service for family planning advice. She was initially dubious about contraception, fearful of its effect on her future fertility. In the end she chose the pill. She required much support to help her persevere with it because of the off/on nature of her relationship with her boyfriend. Every time they had a row she was tempted to throw the pills away. But when they made it up they invariably had sex. Without the pill she would probably have had two children instead of one by the age of eighteen. When the baby was eleven months old Shirley broke off her relationship with John completely, as she had seen him with another girl. She was encouraged to continue with the pill — a wise precaution, in the event. It was not long before she had a new boyfriend, an older man whose wife was chronically ill. It is perhaps not surprising that Shirley, growing up without a father and being rejected by John, should have opted for an older, seemingly more stable person.

This case illustrates the need some girls have to get pregnant to escape an unhappy home, and the precariousness of teenage relationships. It also illustrates their vulnerability to further pregnancies unless sustained support is given with contraception.

The older single mother

Some of the factors which result in pregnancy in the teenage

unmarried mother also apply to the older single woman. How
ever, for some of these older women the decision to have or to
keep a child once pregnancy is discovered may be an attempt to
salvage something for themselves before it is too late as well as
to confirm their femininity and fertility. This may happen when
a relationship of long standing is breaking up or where the man
is already married. Some unmarried older mothers, may, of
course, have made a deliberate conscious choice to get preg
nant and 'go it alone' without a man. Regardless of the moral
view of such behaviour, the burdens both emotional and finan
cial are very heavy unless the mother is supported by her
family.

Divorced and separated

Divorce is becoming commoner in our society; 1 in 4 of all
marriages end in divorce. Teenage marriages are particularly
vulnerable to breakdown.

6 per cent of couples marrying in 1971 under the age of
twenty had divorced by 1975, compared with 2 per cent in the
20–24 age bracket (*Social Trends*, 1977). The young married
couple often face housing difficulties which add to the tension
of marriage: of the 35,000 young couples where the husband
was under twenty only about half had their own home.

The number of separations or couples living apart cannot be
estimated. The risk of unintended pregnancies in this group is
high, as a result of loneliness, isolation and feelings of worth
lessness.

Comparison between unmarried mothers referred for domicili-
ary planning in Haringey

During 1968–1976 400 unmarried mothers (this figure includes
teenage mothers), just under a third of all the cases referred for
domiciliary family planning in Haringey. Reference has already
been made to some of the findings. It must be remembered that
this is not a random sample. Cases were selected for referral by
health visitors or social workers or self-selected for domiciliary
care as they were in special need.

The 2 Greek Cypriot, 3 Indian and 2 mixed parentage and 12
Irish have been included in the British group as their numbers
are small. This group was compared to 264 unmarried mothers
of West Indian origin. It was found that:

1. In well over half of both groups the mothers themselves come from large families (five +).

2. Over 60 per cent of mothers in the 'British' group come from 'broken' homes, through the separation or divorce or death of parents compared to 45 per cent of the West Indian group. Those who themselves were illegitimate were more likely to have been 'in care' if they were British, whereas the illegitimate West Indian girl was often reared in a family setting with a step-parent, usually a stepfather. Only three West Indian girls came into care as a result of being orphans. The rest (11 per cent) came into care in their early teens as being 'beyond parental control', running away from home, etc.

3. There were proportionately more pregnancies among the West Indian group with a larger number of abortions. 69 per cent of the West Indian group had had more than one pregnancy compared to 54 per cent of the British.

4. 44 per cent of the West Indian mothers had different fathers for their pregnancies compared to 30 per cent of the British group.

5. The West Indian mothers tended to have their first conception earlier than the British group, though the difference is not marked.

MENTAL AND EMOTIONAL DIFFICULTIES

Parents under stress

Parents under stress from whatever cause may need help and support with family planning. The stress can be due to:

a) socio-economic factors — poor housing, overcrowding, threats of eviction, shortage of money, debts, unemployment,

b) marital and relationship difficulties, especially where there is violence and the couple are immature;

c) illness, physical and mental, especially where this interferes with work and the care of the children;

d) isolation, loneliness, separation from family and friends;

e) care of several small children, especially if this occurs in poor housing isolated from family and friends.

All these factors can exist together and exacerbate each other. Thus overcrowding and poor housing can worsen marital difficulties. Both can lead to poor care of children or even child abuse where the child becomes the victim of the parents' frustration and misery. In families where violence occurs pregnancy tends to happen either because the man deliberately wants to make the woman pregnant to control her and prevents her using contraception or because he cannot be bothered with contraception. Unfortunately, the violence may be exacerbated as a result of an unplanned pregnancy with the man jealous of the baby (Renvoize 1978). Children themselves can, of course, add to the stress; the fatigue associated with the care of small children can lead to marital difficulties. The children may be neglected and have to be taken into care. This in itself may cause such powerful feelings of hopelessness and failure that the mother allows herself to get pregnant to replace the child(ren) in care. The social worker needs to be sensitive to this aspect of removing children from home.

Depression

High rates of depression were found in women with young children, with the highest rates in working-class women with a child under six (Brown *et al.* 1973, 1975, Richman 1974). The depression was in response to stress — living in flats isolated with small children. Four factors were found to predispose women to developing depression under stress: lack of confiding relationship with husband or boyfriend, not going out to work, having lost their own mother before the age of eleven, and having three or more children under 14 (Richman 1977).

Childbirth itself may contribute to the increased rates of depression in women with small children. In a general practice population study depression was increased five-fold in women in the three months after delivery compared with the rate during pregnancy (Ryle 1961). It is not known whether the depression is the result of hormonal changes or of the tiredness and responsibility associated with the care of a new baby. The depressed woman is at risk from losing control and physically abusing her children. Many of the mothers, both married and unmarried, seen by the Haringey Domiciliary FP Service are depressed. They are usually isolated from family and friends and may live in a tower block or slum conditions with inadequate play space for their children who are always under their feet. The depression is usually associated with apathy so that they are unable to help themselves, and this includes getting family planning advice. Thus such a mother is at risk from becoming unintentionally pregnant.

The following case illustrates the sequence of event

described above and the particular vulnerability of young immature parents.

Mr and Mrs J. were both twenty years old with two small children; one aged thirteen months, the other one month. Mr J. came from a large, easy-going family. He did night work. Mrs J. was the only daughter in a family of three and as such was much doted on and spoiled and not allowed to grow up. She became pregnant before marriage and had to get married. The family lived in a two-room flat on the fourteenth floor of a tower block, away from both their families. Mrs J. hated the flat and became very depressed after the second child (unplanned). Mr J. had to take time off work to take care of Mrs J. and the children. She was afraid to be on her own at nights. He lost his job and found it difficult to find another. Debts began to pile up — worry over this, and tiredness as a result of broken nights with the babies, led to constant bickering. Mr J. started to drink, become violent when drunk and kept threatening to leave.

Mrs J. had been given the oral contraceptive pill by the hospital (enough for 3 months) after the second baby and was advised to get further supplies from her GP. The difficulties were such that Mrs J. was just too tired or too harassed to go to the GP for the pill. She convinced herself that the contraceptive effects of the pill would last for several months after finishing the last packet. Six months after the second baby she was pregnant again. Mr J. left. Mrs J. then abandoned the children and the NSPCC were involved. The children were taken into care. The eldest child was found to have bruises on his arms and legs thought to be caused by the parents. Eventually, the parents returned to the flat and Mrs J. was referred by the health visitor for domiciliary family planning advice. Mrs J. was considering abortion for the unplanned pregnancy. Mr J. was opposed to this. During the first interview with the doctor the bitterness and resentment from both Mr and Mrs J. spilled over. They attacked and blamed each other for their troubles and especially their respective families. Mr J. blamed Mrs J.'s mother and said she had spoilt her and was always interfering. He was against abortion and said she should have the baby. She agreed to have the baby provided he promised not to leave her. Mrs J. had the baby and so had three children under 2½ years. The family needed intensive visiting by both the social services and the domiciliary service. The children were returned to the couple. Eventually the family were rehoused. Support was necessary from both the social services and domiciliary family planning service until the two older children were at school.

Schizophrenia

This affects almost 1 in every 100 people. The incidence in the population is 0.85 per cent. It is the commonest psychiatric disorder. Although treatment has improved to the extent that many patients who have it can now live in the community, it cannot be cured. The outlook is determined by the number of breakdowns — the more there are, the worse the prognosis. Inevitably many such patients, even though they may not have been born into social classes IV and V, end up at the lower end of the social scale since they cannot work regularly.

Women with schizophrenia or whose partners have schizophrenia may need careful contraceptive counselling. The pill and mechanical methods may not be suitable because, during a breakdown, the woman may forget to use it. Care is needed during a breakdown since the woman may get paranoid ideas about the contraceptive method controlling her and making her ill.

'Personality disorders' (pathological personality-psychopathic disorders)

These are difficult to define. 'Most psychiatrists prefer to assert that they can recognise psychopathic disorder more easily than they can define it' (Tredgold & Wolff 1970). Some people who have personality disorders seem to manage their lives reasonably well except for occasional eccentric and bizarre behaviour. They are not necessarily unintelligent. Others manifest bizarre, unpredictable and impulsive behaviour accompanied by violence. Perhaps these should be classified as having psychopathic traits in that their behaviour is often callous. When a woman is affected in this way she may embark on repeated pregnancies in a thoughtless and careless way that may prove impossible to control, though the problem she creates with her family may involve all the social agencies.

Just under 1 per cent of all women (1,500) referred to the Haringey Domiciliary Family Planning Service during 1968—76 could be so characterised. Although the families associated with the women had many problems (so called multi-problem families), this is not to say that the parents of all multi-problem families have personality disorders or psychopathic traits. It is necessary to make this distinction since the term 'multi-problem family' has come to be used almost as a generic term, lumping together families where the reasons for the problems may be quite disparate. Men, of course, may also have pathological personalities. Their behaviour often brings them into conflict with the law. Their relationship with women may be hostile and though superficially charming their hostility may lead them to repeatedly impregnate their wives or girlfriends without concern for their health and wellbeing.

Clinical experience indicates that women with such personality disorders are erratic users of contraception. They have required intensive and not always successful visiting by the domiciliary service. The women, though superficially friendly, lack real warmth and it is difficult to make a relationship with them of any depth. They can be depressing to work with and often make the worker feel both inadequate and devalued. Focusing on family spacing rather than limitation may be a more realistic aim with such families.

LARGE FAMILIES
(Family size 5 or more children)

As we have seen earlier, many large families are large not because the parents desire it but because it just 'happens'. Such families tend to be found among the lower socio-economic groups. There is also a preponderance of large families among poor Catholics, particularly Scots and Irish, West Indians who emigrated to England in the 1950s, and Asians from the Indian subcontinent. 7.2 per cent of the families referred to the Haringey Domiciliary Service during 1968–76 had five or more children (112 families out of 1,500).

Some parents of large families tend to become fatalistic and apathetic about their situation and feel that nothing will work for them. They share many of the attitudes described by Rainwater (see Chapter 9). The husband may be reluctant to use precautions himself, though he is not necessarily opposed to the idea of family planning. The woman in such a situation may feel too embarrassed to seek help and only when life really gets desperate does she demand that the doctor at hospital after her last confinement 'do something'. A recent study (Bone 1978) has shown that women who had had more pregnancies than average had never used contraception or had used it sporadically.

Although some mothers of large families can see no rôle for themselves other than that of mother, experience from the Haringey Domiciliary Service shows that they often do not produce as many children as their own mothers. This shows that they have attempted (albeit with limited success) to limit their own family size.

Some mothers, out of deep inner needs due to their own lack of mothering, have large families to give them significance and self-esteem. Only bad obstetric experience may cause them to limit their fertility. One such was Rose. She was the illegitimate child of a soldier and had been adopted by a couple who brought her up as an only child. She felt lonely and rejected as a child and was determined to have a large family to give her the love and companionship that she felt she had lacked. She married a man who had mild epilepsy and worked as a warehouseman. She had her first child at fifteen before getting married and then had a total of nine children in ten years. One of her children died in infancy. She was referred for domiciliary family planning by her health visitor. She was then twenty-seven years old. Rose found something wrong with all the methods, and on further discussion revealed that she loved babies; they made her feel alive. Her husband was not so sanguine and was anxious to be sterilised. Rose refused to sign the consent form. She then went on to have her tenth and had a bad pregnancy. That baby also died. Rose then agreed to let her husband have the operation. When seen in the street a few years later, she said she still 'fancied a baby' but felt she had had enough.

Whether couples have large families through chance or as a deliberate policy, it seems as though a 'breaking-point' is reached for most of them, either as a result of poor health or straitened resources, emotional and material or both, and they do end up wanting contraceptive help, usually in the form of sterilisation.

THE HANDICAPPED

As mentioned in Chapter 3, attitudes towards the personal and sexual needs of the handicapped are changing, not least among the handicapped themselves. Thus handicapped people want to lead as normal a life as possible and that may mean getting married and having children. In order to realise this, considerable support from both the family and the community may be necessary. Contraceptive and genetic counselling have an important role in preventing the individual or couple being strained beyond their physical or emotional resources. The normal couple who have had a handicapped child are also in need of such counselling to prevent their being overwhelmed by the birth of another handicapped child. Genetic counselling is available through large paediatric departments. Referral is usually through the GP. Since the degree of disability can vary enormously, each person or couple must be counselled within the limits of the disability. Help may need to be brought to the couple since restricted mobility is often a feature of handicapped life — clinics may have steps, for example, that the handicapped cannot climb. Thus referral to a domiciliary family planning service (where it exists) may be appropriate. Failing this the social worker may need to take the couple to a suitable clinic.

The physically handicapped

Contraception may be unnecessary for those whose handicap also affects sexual function, particularly for the man who cannot obtain or sustain an erection and/or who may be infertile (spinal cord injury, spina bifida and multiple sclerosis in its advanced stages). Women suffering from these disorders may be able to become pregnant. The choice of contraceptive can be difficult since the woman needs to be protected against infection. The mechanical methods may be inadvisable because of this. The coil will need very careful supervision since any pelvic infection may go undetected in a woman with little pelvic sensation. The pill may prove hazardous for those with circulatory problems because of the risk of thrombosis. However, pregnancy itself carries similar risks of pelvic and urinary infection and thrombosis. Thus, where the couple opt not to have children or decide their family is complete, sterilisation may be the answer. It is safer, for example, to be sterilised than to take the pill for twenty years or have a coil fitted and run the risk of pregnancy which may need to be terminated.

Care of multiple sclerosis

Mrs K. was twenty-two years old, a pretty girl who developed multiple sclerosis after her first pregnancy. Her second pregnancy resulted in twins. After their birth she was bedridden, her legs and arms were weak and she became incontinent. After many months, during which time her children were in care, she improved to the extent of being able to walk round the bed. It took six months for her to accept that she had multiple sclerosis and that her future health would be uncertain with remissions and exacerbations. During remissions she would be almost her normal self but during the exacerbations she could become paralysed and incapacitated. Her husband, initially afraid of the idea of a vasectomy, later decided he would get it done. Mrs K., once the implications of her illness had really been understood and accepted, opted for sterilisation. She did not want more children and did not want to take the pill for years. She also felt that since she was the partner with the illness and she might die sooner than her husband, who might wish to remarry, it was really her decision. A year after the birth of the twins she was sterilised. She and her husband had been extremely fertile and had had three children in two years.

The blind

It may be difficult for the blind person to imagine the size of the female genital organs and examinations can be bewildering and frightening unless care is taken to explain what is being done. The mechanical methods such as the cap or sheath are not very suitable and the pill, an injectable hormone such as Depoprovera, and the coil are probably the best methods. The coil may prove unacceptable if it causes heavy and irregular periods.

Mrs O. is twenty-two years of age. She is totally blind and has been so since birth. She was one of a large family and her blindness was caused by an excess of oxygen given to her as a premature baby. Her mother died when she was very young and so she and her brothers and sisters went into care. She met her husband, who is partially blind, on a training course. He is twenty-four. They had one child soon after marriage, delivered by caesarean as Mrs O. has a small pelvis. She became very depressed after the birth and was unable to care for the baby who went into care for six months. She had horrific fantasies about the operation and wanted to talk about it repeatedly and to know exactly what was done step by step. She opted to take the pill and managed to take it well. She was visited every month, initially by the domiciliary service. There would be occasional panic when her pills got lost. She stopped the pill after two years and then had another child, also by caesarean, and she has returned to the pill. Recently her eldest child, a little girl, who is sighted, took her pills and Mrs O. was very distressed because she could not find out whether she had eaten them. This made her decide to have a coil instead. She plans to have one more child and then be sterilised.

The mentally handicapped

The mentally handicapped, unaffected by physical handicaps, do not usually have any problems with sexual functioning or fertility. Hence there is often anxiety surrounding mentally handicapped girls who may be at risk of exploitation and may not be able to cope responsibly with their sexuality.

The handicapped may find the mechanical methods and the pill too difficult to cope with and so the best methods at present available are probably the IUD, the intramuscular injection Depoprovera and sterilisation. However, these methods need careful explanation and the girl needs preparation before a referral to a clinic or doctor. If she is taken to a clinic without such preparation she may be too shocked to accept the fitting of a coil and her fear may be such that she refused to go to the clinic or doctor again. The helper must be careful to explain in simple terms as much as, but no more than, he or she thinks the handicapped person will understand. If explanations are too detailed the handicapped person may be bewildered or terrified, or both. The mother of a handicapped daughter may be ashamed to bring her to the clinic or she may bring her without explaining to her what it is for.

The management of mentally handicapped girls may be difficult if they are without the support of their families and alone in the city. Some are tempted into prostitution. Others are at risk from repeated pregnancies which may overwhelm their capabilities.

Patsy is nineteen, English, and mentally handicapped. She is overweight. She got pregnant at sixteen and had to get married. She herself was an only child and illegitimate. A year later a

second pregnancy occurred. When she got pregnant the thir
time shortly afterwards she demanded an abortion. By th
time her marriage had broken down and her husband had le
her. She was a poor housekeeper and her house was perpetu
ally dirty. She liked a 'good time' and men to make a fuss ϲ
her. One night she went off to a dance leaving her two sma
children alone. The police found the oldest, aged three, wande
ing in the road. The children were taken into care. Patsy fell
love with a married man. He had recently come out of priso
Patsy has had a baby by him. Although now fitted with a co
Patsy says she wants 'lots of babies'. Her children are all on th
'at risk' register as bruises have repeatedly been found on ther

It is not suggested that all mentally handicapped women hav
such tragic lives and fail to care for their children. Some ϲ
cope, given outside support, *provided they do not have tϲ
many children too quickly*.

Since the mentally handicapped are often deterred by tʰ
new and unfamiliar, the domiciliary service (where it exisϮ
may be the most acceptable way of providing family planniɴ
help.

14
The Influence of Religion and Culture

All the great religions of the world have been and still are to a large extent pro-natalist, anti-abortion and anti-sterilisation. However, attitudes are gradually being modified so that only the very strict adherents of a particular religion will condemn any use of contraception. Thus when advising couples from other countries who live in Britain about contraception, it is important to take account of their religious background and the extent to which they accept or reject their religious teaching as far as birth control, abortion and sterilisation are concerned. These can be openly acknowledged in the following way by a comment such as, 'I know that you are Moslem (Catholic etc.) and that the decision about birth control, abortion etc. may be a difficult one. What do you feel about this?' This allows the individual or couple either to reject any advice on the basis that it is against their religion or to admit how far they go along with the teachings of their religion regarding family planning and related matters.

Women born in other countries, particularly India, Pakistan and the West Indies, tend to want larger families than those born in Britain (Cartwright 1976). This does not mean that they are opposed to family planning or birth control provided the professional helper is sensitive to their beliefs and values. The immigrant families are found usually in the cities — London and in the Midlands — where they may live in poor, overcrowded conditions. Despite this, the close-knit extended-family pattern of many of the immigrant families may be supportive to such an extent that very little use is made of the social worker or social services.

Immigrants have usually come to Britain because of job opportunities and for a better future for their children. They may also have come as refugees from countries going through political turmoil such as the East African Asians and Greek Cypriots. There is a tendency to lump all immigrants together without trying to understand or appreciate their very different traditions and ways of living.

CATHOLICISM

Catholicism is pro-natalist and sex tends to be seen solely in reproductive terms. The papal encyclical *Humanae Vitae* (1968) is opposed to all forms of contraception except for the rhythm or safe period. Catholicism is not opposed to family planning in its literal sense but relies more on self-control and abstinence to achieve this. Abortion and sterilisation are opposed. The Church's teaching regarding contraception together with its attitudes towards sex can make the continued use of contraception difficult.

Thus the ambivalence and conflict experienced by Catholic women may lead to frequent complaints about the method of birth control. These should be explored, and not accepted at face value. Reliance is often placed on withdrawal since this does not necessitate public admission of the use of birth control, and interestingly it may not be regarded as such by the women.

However, although Catholic couples tend to want and have larger families than other couples seen in both American and British fertility studies (Woolf 1972, Cartwright 1976), nevertheless, all the methods of birth control are used and abortion itself is resorted to when a woman cannot face another pregnancy. Also, although contraception is not used, once a woman has the number of children she feels she can adequately cope with she may well request sterilisation. This has been seen repeatedly among Catholic women referred to the Haringey domiciliary service.

Some priests are leaving the decision concerning the use of birth control methods (other than the rhythm method) to the conscience of the woman or couple concerned.

Irish Catholics

A special reference to Irish Catholics is made here since Catholicism as practised in Ireland tends to be stricter than that in England. The papal encyclical *Humanae Vitae* has more force in Ireland than England. The first family planning clinic opened in Dublin in 1969 was called the Fertility Guidance Clinic There are now eight family planning clinics in Ireland and they are openly called Family Planning Clinics. Many family doctors prescribe the pill for 'menstrual irregularities'. There has been a regular contraceptive trade between Northern Ireland and Eire.

Despite the emphasis on modesty and prohibitions against premarital sex, pregnancy before marriage does occur. The girls often come to England either to have an abortion or to have the baby so that their families will not discover that they are pregnant.

The modesty and shame surrounding sex prevent many Irish women going to clinics or their GPs (because they are men) for advice. The vaginal examination is particularly disliked and feared. Its value lies both in revealing sexual difficulties and helping the woman accept her own body. Husbands may similarly be too embarrassed to buy the sheaths. They may hide this by saying that 'It's against my religion' but may use the sheaths if they are sent through the post. If the man is too embarrassed to buy the sheath or refuses to use it, the onus is then put on the woman and, as mentioned earlier, this may prove too much for her. Thus as most couples do not want repeated pregnancies, excuses are made by the woman to avoid sex. The ensuing arguments often result in the man seeking solace in drink.

Mrs B. was twenty-eight years old and had seven children, one every year since 1961. She had a bad seventh pregnancy with toxaemia (high blood pressure) and sterilisation was recommended. Her husband refused to sign the consent form, not out of malice but because he was afraid that she would die under the anaesthetic and he would be held responsible. For a year afterwards they lived a cat-and-dog life. They had two bedrooms, Mrs B. sleeping in one with the seven children and Mr B. in the other. This was their method of birth control. Mr B. used to drink heavily every Saturday night and attempt to have intercourse. Mrs B. was referred for domiciliary help. The coil was chosen and eight years later there have been no more pregnancies. They have been rehoused and Mrs B. looks years younger. One of Mrs B.'s frequent comments is, 'If only I'd known about family planning sooner I wouldn't have had all these children, much as I love them now'.

The social worker should not be deterred by official Catholic attitudes to birth control from discussing contraception with Catholic clients. Most will welcome it, provided it is done with sensitivity and tact.

HINDUISM

Families practising the Hindu religion come from India, East Africa and the West Indies. Those families which adhere strongly to the religion are more likely to come from India. Families from India tend to be poor, illiterate and from villages (80 per cent of the Indian population live in villages). The man may speak English to a limited extent; the woman rarely can. The Indians who migrated to East Africa tended to become involved in commercial interests. They are more educated and literate and have adopted a more Western style of living, as have the Indian West Indians.

The Hindu religion is one of the oldest in the world. It involves the worship of many gods and goddesses. Hindus outside India do not build temples but practise their religion at home. There is belief in the transmigration of souls. Traditional Hinduism upholds the division of society into castes. There are four main castes but many subcastes. Contact and marriage between castes is forbidden. There is fear of pollution. All bodily discharges are considered polluting, especially faeces. The untouchables (Harijans), or lowest caste, are those whose job it is to remove human faeces. The caste system does not now have legal sanction and its influence is being modified.

It is a male-dominated society and the role of the woman is subservient. Once married she becomes incorporated within her husband's family which includes his parents, uncles, aunts, brothers and their families. She must respect the wishes of her husband's relatives, particularly his mother's, more than her own. Her husband must be the centre of all her activities and she must never raise a word against him.

Marriage Marriages are arranged. Marriages by choice (*qandharva*) are considered improper and undesirable. Marriage is a social duty towards the family and the community and the individual's need of personal happiness is not recognised (Kapadia 1966). Marriage has a threefold purpose:

(1) To lead the good life, *dharma*. This involves daily religious duties to be performed by the husband with his wife before the sacred fire kindled in the home at the time of marriage by the priest or brahmin. This is the most important purpose of marriage.

(2) Procreation, especially of a son. A son is needed to say prayers and ensure the survival of the father in the next world. The word for son is *putra* which literally means he who saves

from hell (*put*). Thus large families might result in the effort to obtain a son.

(3) *Sex (Kāma).* The bride must be a virgin as this adds to the honour of the marriage. The girl also has to have a dowry. Thus girls are an economic liability. One way of obtaining dowries for daughters was by marrying off sons and using the daughter-in-laws' dowries. Hindu marriage is a sacrament, complete only on the performance of special rites by the priest. As such it is irrevocable even if one of the partners is unfaithful. It has a further significance for both the man and the woman. For the man it is one of several sacraments performed during the course of his life. For the woman it is essential as it is the only sacrament that can be performed for her. Fidelity of both partners is expected. The boy and girl do not meet before marriage, though they may do so in England. Once a woman has produced a son, her status is improved and the bond between the mother and her eldest son is often very close. She will subsequently in her turn be able to exercise power over her daughter-in-law. Children are indulged in Indian families and there are many women within the family to care for them. There is little emphasis on developing self-reliance in the child or treating him as an individual person (Lannoy 1971). The reasons for this are probably twofold: the greater importance of the family as opposed to the individual, and the fact that one in ten children die in the Indian villages. This has significance when advising such mothers about contraception, for their experience of life is that because all the children a woman has do not survive, one must have many to ensure the survival of a few, especially a son. It will take time for Indian mothers in England to realise that most if not all the children they have here will survive. Children are breast-fed till two years of age (used also as a means of contraception) and may sleep with the mother until five years.

Contraception Attitudes to this will be influenced by economic and educational status — the more educated the couple, the greater the acceptance of contraception. With the less educated and poorer families family planning advice will achieve greater success if the husband is involved. Women tend to be shy and modest and reluctant to allow a vaginal examination, particularly by a male doctor.

Sometimes the man wants to take charge and he will use the sheath. The coil may not be favoured since it causes heavy periods and the woman is unclean when menstruating and not allowed to cook for the family. Some women with large families choose sterilisation when it is offered to them. The main fear of the men in this situation is that the sterilisation should not make her 'sick'. The pill usually poses more problems as it is often difficult for the woman to understand how it works; therefore, she may fail to take it every day. As with most communities, if a friend or relative is using a method successfully then this is the greatest incentive for the woman to choose that particular method. Thus where one woman has had success she will bring her female relations along to the clinic.

Language may be a barrier. Leaflets in Urdu, Punjabi and Bengali are available from the Family Planning Association. Several drug firms also produce leaflets.

ISLAM

The majority of the families from Pakistan and Bangladesh (formerly East Pakistan) are Moslem. They tend to be poor, illiterate and from villages. Some Asian families from East Africa are Moslem. They (like the Hindu families) are usually more educated and literate. Turkish Cypriots are also Moslem, but they will be considered later with the Greek Cypriots, as, despite different religions, they share similar attitudes towards marriage and contraception. (Strict religious observance is more likely to be found among Pakistani and Bangladeshi (they tend to have larger families) than among Turkish Cypriot and East African families. Islam literally means submission to the Will of Allah or God. It is a way of life which lays down principles and values on which different aspects of individual and social life are organised. Moslems are meant to pray five times a day and to practise fasting for one month (Ramadan) in the year. The family is the central institution. The man is the head of the household though he may have to defer to an older male head of the whole family. This happens particularly among Pakistani and Bangladeshi families. Marriages are arranged. In well-to-do families there is a tendency to marry within the family, i.e. first cousin marriage. Dowries have to be found for daughters. However, a special bride price is paid (the *Mahr*) to the bride by the bridegroom before he has intercourse with her. Sometimes the full bride price is only paid when the husband dies or divorces his wife. The bride must be a virgin. Fidelity is expected of the wife, who can be divorced if she is unfaithful. Marriage is only recognised after a religious ceremony performed in the bride's house. It must not be consummated until this is performed. Among poorer families marriages are arranged when the girl is prepubertal.

Although equal in Moslem law and practice, women are considered inferior to men. The woman's life is centred on the home and she sees herself, and is seen, principally in the rôles of wife and mother. She is expected to be respectful and obedient towards her husband. She may only participate in family decisions when she is older. The family is an extended one and members are supposed to be responsible for each other. Sex is for procreation. A husband's love for his wife is believed to be demonstrated by the number of children she has. Birth control is discouraged except for medical reasons. Abortion and sterilisation are prohibited. Intercourse is forbidden during menstruation as the woman is considered unclean. She cannot go to the mosque to pray or touch the *Qu'ran* when menstruating. Thus the IUD may not be acceptable if it produces prolonged periods. Women tend to be modest and reserved and dislike vaginal examinations or touching themselves, hence the cap or pessaries may not be acceptable.

For some Asian families from Pakistan, India and Bangladesh, 'home' is still in those countries and connections are assiduously maintained. Some young people born here are being sent 'home' at puberty so that marriages can be arranged there.

FAMILIES FROM CYPRUS

Cyprus was a British colony from 1875 until 1960. The population consists of 80 per cent Greek Cypriot and 20 per cent Turkish Cypriot. Before the British took over Cyprus it belonged to Turkey for nearly four hundred years.

Greek Cypriot

The bulk of Greek Cypriot families came to England in the 1950s and settled mainly in North London. The largest population of Greek Cypriots live in the London Borough of Haringey. A further influx of families occurred after Turkey invaded Cyprus in 1974. These refugees were incorporated into the existing Greek families. Greek Cypriots are Christian and belong to the Greek Orthodox faith.

It is a male-dominated society. The family is important and members of it are expected to help each other. Marriages are arranged, though this may occur to a lesser extent for the young born in Britain. Virginity is highly valued and Greek girls are expected to be virgins when they marry. Proof may be sought in blood-stained sheets on the wedding night. Any girl with a rumour of a reputation will find it difficult to marry within the community. There is a double standard of morality, and men are allowed sexual experience before marriage either with prostitutes or with girls from other nationalities. Boys are more valued than girls since a dowry has to be found for the latter when they marry. The Greek Orthodox faith is not opposed to contraception and the men usually either practise withdrawal or use the sheath. Some of the women born here and who can read English are now using the pill and coil. The Greek couples rarely want or intend to have a large family. Those couples referred for domiciliary FP in Haringey have on an average three children. They are referred usually because there is a language difficulty.

Turkish Cypriot

Turkish families are mainly found in London, particularly North London. They are Moslem, though tend to be less religious than Arabs or Pakistanis. Again it is a male-dominated society. Marriages are arranged (couples may talk to each other before marriage, but not go out together). Dowries have to be found for daughters. Sons are more valued. There is no sex education in the home. Usually the men will take charge of contraception, using the sheath or withdrawal, though the younger women, particularly those born here, are adopting the pill and coil. The young people do not intend or want large families, though they may belong to them. Those Turkish Cypriot families referred for domiciliary FP advice in Haringey tend to be larger than the Greek Cypriot. This usually comes about because the man will not take responsibility for contraception and the woman, too shy and speaking poor English, is afraid to go to the clinics or her GP.

All the cultural groups so far examined, apart from the Irish, have several common features. They are patriarchal and male-dominated and stress is placed on virginity before marriage, particularly for the women. Thus daughters are closely guarded and may not be allowed to go out in the evening without a chaperone. Fertility is important because these families come from areas where there is a high infant mortality rate. Also they are from agricultural communities where children are seen as helping hands and an insurance for old age. It is possible that the families who emigrate do so because they are more adventuresome and less rigidly adherent to their own cultural norms. Nevertheless, many of the old patterns are recreated in Britain. Cheetham (1972) noted that social workers are more likely to find themselves working with the children of immigrant families who find themselves torn between two cultures and owing allegiance to neither. Indications of this have occurred already. In Haringey there have been two suicides of teenage girls (one Greek and one Turkish) who felt constrained by their families. They were not permitted to bring friends home or go out in the evening, even with girl friends. Such was the anxiety of the parents concerning their daughters' virginity that they saw any manifestation of independence as a threat that must be guarded against at all costs. This may seem abhorrent to English people used to greater individual freedom, but the 'reputation', or as one Greek father put it, the 'respect', of the girls is of paramount importance, or they will become outcasts in their communities. These conflicts between the parents' way of life and that of their friends is seen more clearly in school and particularly in teaching about sexual matters. Greek, Turkish and Asian girls tend to be shy and modest and easily shocked. They know about the significance of virginity — that much 'sex education' is given at home — but they have all kinds of fantasies about what will happen on their wedding night and how much they will bleed and the pain involved in intercourse. Frequent questions asked are, 'Can a tampax destroy virginity?', 'If you don't bleed on your wedding night are you still a virgin?' Some in anxiety arrange their weddings to coincide with their periods.

WEST INDIAN FAMILIES

Although at first glance it may appear irrelevant to West Indian family life in Britain (especially as this is undergoing change) to look at that in the West Indies, certain attitudes particularly with regard to sex, marriage and illegitimacy cannot be understood without doing so. Furthermore, since these are, to quote

Hiro (1971) 'rooted in the historical experience of slavery' this too will be touched upon here. There is a risk of over-simplification obviously in dealing with such a complex subject in a short space so readers are referred to other works (see list of Useful Books, p. 321–2).

Under slavery women were encouraged to produce children but were forbidden to marry. Both they and their children and, of course, the fathers were the sole responsibility of the slave owner. Thus the father's place was never secure. He was not the source of protection and provision for the mother and her children. The slave owner himself often took concubines, and was responsible for the children. This led to an improved social status. From these came the 'coloured' middle class that adopted the values of white society in regard to occupation, marriage and illegitimacy.

Two studies, one sociological (Clarke 1957) and one on fertility (Blake 1961), have thrown light on West Indian family life particularly as regards sexual attitudes, common law unions, illegitimacy and marriage. Henriques (himself West Indian) (1956) also provides useful insight. However, the conclusions he draws about what Jamaicans want and why they behave the way they do, are *not* from actual data but by inference from behaviour. This has met with criticism from both Clarke and Blake. Clarke, for example, showed that the people she talked to were well aware of the difference between common law marriage and legal marriage (denied by Henriques) and do not confuse the two. Legal marriage is considered a very serious matter with obligations on the husband to support his wife and their children and her 'outside' children (children by another man before marriage). Common law marriages do not bring such obligations nor social status to the women, though they are better than sexual unions without cohabitation. Faithfulness is expected in marriage and in cohabitation, though with the latter either partner is free to separate. Since marriage requires that the man supports the wife it cannot be entered into lightly. He must have a house and land. Thus marriage tends to occur later in a couple's life. Common law marriage does not necessarily lead to marriage and illegitimacy is not a social stigma.

The three communities studied by Clarke had different attitudes to sex, procreation and cohabitation. These were dependent on economic status. The group which was comprised of farmers who owned their own land was the most stable with marriage as the norm. The father tended to be strict and very much in charge of the family. In the second group, where families lived on smallholdings, conjugal relationships were the norm. In the third group, which was the poorest where the men worked as farm labourers, sexual unions were more usual than marriage or cohabitation. Men boasted about their sexual prowess and the number of children they had fathered. Precocious sexual behaviour in adolescent boys was much admired and sexual activity was regarded as 'natural'. It was considered unnatural for the woman not to have a child. 'A child is God's gift' and 'nothing should be done to prevent the birth of the child'. A barren woman was called a mule. It was considered that a woman was only a real woman after bearing a child. There is a common belief (prevalent among some West Indians in Britain) that a man knows in the act of coitus that he has impregnated the woman. The man does not necessarily accept any of the obligations and duties of parenthood. This is considered a woman's responsibility.

Blake (1961) confirmed these findings. She also found that girls were kept in ignorance about sex and fear was expressed that if the girl knew about sex she would go and experiment. Parents seemed to have little faith in the children developing inner controls and so a strict authoritarian control was exerted by the parents (or the mother if she was alone). This is seen among West Indian families in Britain where parents are so fearful of their daughters becoming pregnant that they are not allowed out. Sometimes a girl rebels against this and runs away. She is then likely to come to the notice of the social services. The parents often express the view that they cannot 'chastise', i.e. beat, their children in Britain as they would do back home.

Clarke and Blake both found that if a girl did get pregnant the man was not held responsible and the pregnancy was treated in four almost ritualised stages. First, the girl had sex surreptitiously and once the pregnancy was discovered it was greeted with noisy scolding. The girl was then beaten and turned out of the house; she usually then went to a neighbour or kinswoman who interceded with the mother. The girl was then taken back and the mother might take care of the child. The girl might not have further sexual relations for some time. Then a new sexual union might occur that might lead to another pregnancy. One pattern is for such a girl to have several children by different men in the vain hope that one of them may support her and her children. The more children she has the less chance there is of marriage. Another pattern is for sexual union to lead to cohabitation or common law marriage. There is no security attached to this and there are few mutual obligations. Is this early sexual experimentation related to attitudes towards sex and fertility? Blake thinks there is no pressure on the girls to prove their fertility since parents do want their daughters to marry but feel they are too immature till their twenties. The men are 'footloose' and there are no social sanctions against their having intercourse. They are not forced to marry their pregnant sweethearts and, indeed, marriage for the poor has few rewards. Thus among the poor families the child learns that children are a woman's concern. The relationship with father is usually ambivalent.

Clarke and Blake both found that the men were against birth control. It must be remembered that only the sheath and pessaries were then available. Blake concluded that if birth control was used by the girl *before* she had borne any illegitimate children and if there were fewer children in marriage the men would be encouraged to marry earlier. However, it would seem obvious that improved economic opportunities would have similar consequences.

How far are these patterns of behaviour with regard to premarital sex and pregnancy being seen in Britain? Clinical experience would seem to indicate that among some young West Indians, particularly those who are unemployed and with few opportunities, these patterns are being repeated. Whereas in the West Indies a neighbour or kinswoman would intercede when a pregnancy occurred and the mother would then look after the child, the social services may be asked by the girl and her family for support and help. In Britain the mother herself is often working and may not be in a position to care for the child.

The West Indian Family in Britain

The older West Indian family

The bulk of the West Indian families came to England in the 1950s and early sixties. They felt a particular affinity and closeness to Britain, not only because they shared a common language but because teaching in West Indian schools was mainly about Britain. Hence their dismay and bewilderment when they experienced prejudice and rejection in their search for jobs and houses (Hiro 1971). The men were usually skilled or semi-skilled workers. Once established, they sent for their wives and children. This might include the 'outside' children. The families tended to be large with 6–10 children. Religion plays a strong part in family life, discipline of the children is strict and unquestioning obedience is expected. Education is seen as vitally important and West Indian parents are ambitious for their children.

As noted earlier, the married man is expected to support his wife and children and the woman should not work. In England, however, the wife usually does go to work because of the greater financial pressures. Commonly, the woman works in a hospital as a ward orderly or state enrolled nurse or in a factory. The couple usually work hard, often unsocial hours so that the husband and wife may not see much of each other. Where the woman stays at home she may feel ambivalent towards her husband's independence and want a more equal relationship. The husband may resent this. There may be considerable friction between the husband and his step-children. Many such families were referred for domiciliary family planning advice in Haringey in the late sixties and early seventies. Couples tended to rely on withdrawal or vaginal pessaries such as gynomin to control their fertility. Most of the women were keen to adopt family planning. Many felt they had enough children and requested sterilisation for themselves.

Mrs F. was a typical example of the women seen by the service at that time. She and her husband came from St Kitts to England in 1964. Mr F. was a fitter's mate. They married in 1955 and had their first child soon after when Mrs F. was eighteen. She had nine children in thirteen years; one child died in infancy. Seven of the children were born in the West Indies. Mr F. practised (not very successfully) 'discharging', i.e. withdrawal. After the ninth child Mrs F. requested sterilisation and this was performed. She was thirty-two.

Some of these mothers were referred to the domiciliary service pregnant and requesting termination and sterilisation, which is contrary to the idea that abortion is never considered by West Indians. 'Her womb is a graveyard' is a West Indian (male) expression for a woman who has had an abortion.

West Indian teenage girls

Girls born in the West Indies As mentioned before, once the West Indian couple had settled in England they sent for their children who had been left behind with the grandmother (usually the mother's mother). By the time they arrived, the couple often had several more children. The children who were brought from the West Indies had an average age of 8–9 years. The shock and bewilderment and sense of estrangement that they felt on arriving in a new country, meeting people who called themselves Mummy and Daddy, whom they neither knew nor recognised (since many parents had left when their offspring were 2–3 years old) was such that many have not even now fully recovered from it. Boys and girls have recounted how this strange person called Mummy asked them to kiss her and how reluctant they felt to do so. Often petted and indulged by grandparents, these children now had to compete with new and unknown siblings for parental affection. They were also expected to look after these siblings. The resentment and hostility grew until in their teenage years the only answer seemed to be to escape. The parents for their part were equally bewildered. Their children seemed difficult to manage, defiant and unloving, spiteful to their brothers and sisters. Added to all this was the poor adjustment by some of these children to school, and so their failure to achieve any academic success was a further source of irritation and disappointment to the parents. With the teens the resentment of the children often turned to open hostility and some of the youngsters ran away from home. Some of the girls saw pregnancy as a solution to their difficulties, a means of getting their own flat and an independent life of their own. The helping professions tended to see this as solely a cultural phenomenon without seeming to appreciate the added stress on these young people.

Girls born in England Some teenage girls who are born in England may also follow a similar pattern of getting pregnant at an early age, much to their parents' displeasure. With some girls cultural factors play the strongest part; with others personal factors and with yet others, both in a complex mixture. Some pregnancies in the early teens, as with other young people will be the result of ignorance and reluctance to obtain advice.

One such was Andrea born in 1960, the youngest of five children. She became pregnant at thirteen by a boy of nineteen. Mother, when she discovered the pregnancy, went to the local social services to find out how to arrange an abortion. She was ambitious for her daughter and wanted her to continue with her studies. The abortion was performed and Andrea had a coil fitted. She was then referred to the domiciliary service by the hospital social worker for follow-up. For about a year an uneasy relationship existed between mother and daughter with mother suspicious of her daughter and not letting her go out, and Andrea resentful at being kept in and treated 'like a child'. Five years later Andrea has a new boy friend and is working for her Advanced Levels with a chance to go to university.

However, some mothers take the view that if their daughter does become pregnant as a teenager then she should have the baby and that this will be 'her lesson' even if the girl herself wants an abortion. In these situations the mother may also refuse to allow her daughter to use contraception, hoping thereby to control her sexual activities. Contraception is seen as a licence to have sex. Where the girl is involved with the social services this can pose a difficult problem.

Illustrative case: parental refusal of abortion

Marcia was a fifteen-year-old West Indian girl under a Section 1 Care Order. She had been put into care as being beyond parental control. Mother was unmarried with four other children, the eldest being in the West Indies. She had latterly become an extremely keen churchgoer and was very strict with Marcia. They had never got on and now there were continual conflicts about clothes and staying out late. In the end Marcia ran away from home. It was discovered that when Marcia came into care she had contracted gonorrhoea and was pregnant. Marcia wanted an abortion.

The social worker was faced with the task of telling mother about the pregnancy, a task made more difficult by the fact that Marcia's mother was a proud and rigid woman. She worked very hard and had managed to provide a good home for her children. She was very bitter about Marcia's behaviour and saw her as ungrateful. When told about the pregnancy Marcia's mother became extremely angry. She said Marcia was wicked and she must have the baby to 'learn her lesson'. She refused under any circumstances to give her consent to an abortion. An attempt was then made to talk about her own pregnancies. With difficulty it was ascertained that her first pregnancy had occurred during her own teens and that this child had been left with her parents. She then came to Britain to do her nursing training but had to give this up as she became pregnant a second time (with Marcia). Marcia's father had abandoned her during pregnancy. Thus the reasons for her past resentment against Marcia became clear. The social worker remarked how disappointed she must have felt when she had to give up her nursing and wondered whether some of the anger she felt towards. Marcia was because of that early disappointment. The mother made no comment but there was a change in her attitude. While still refusing to give her consent to the abortion (now saying that it was against her religion), she agreed to 'the welfare' doing what was best. The daughter was seen by both a psychiatrist and a gynaecologist who agreed that she should have an abortion. This was done. The mother at first refused to see her daughter. Eventually they became reconciled, though the daughter lives in a hostel. She is now studying for her Ordinary Levels.

This case illustrates a number of other issues besides parental refusal. For the West Indian mother, illegitimacy of itself is no disgrace (though this should not be taken to mean that the mother is pleased to see her teenage daughter pregnant). This is often allied to a fatalistic attitude — what's done is done — consequent upon past unfulfilled hopes and ambitions, as in Marcia's mother's case. It also illustrates how West Indian teenagers, like other teenagers (discussed earlier), may become pregnant to draw attention to other problems — in Marcia's case, her feelings of being unloved and resented.

Attitudes to fertility

For yet other girls faced with pregnancy there may be a fear that abortion will damage their fertility. Thus they will go through with the pregnancy even though they do not want a child, despite opposition from both parents and the boyfriend. The reason for this is that the ability to produce a child is an insurance for a future relationship. The girl fears that if she is unable to have a child no man will want her or will stay with her. Thus she may not expect a man to be interested in her as a person but only as a woman who can bear children.

Some girls who get pregnant have the baby to escape from a difficult or unhappy home situation. They say that their mothers will not accept them as adults until they have had a child. The child thus confers status and authority. Sometimes the boyfriend will insist that the girl continues with a pregnancy. Some young men belonging to the Rastafarian sect are opposing the use of contraception. It is unfortunate that the search for an identity, so necessary for young men, who feel excluded from the wider society, is allied to preventing women taking control of their fertility. The high unemployment among West Indian boys leads to loss of self esteem and one way of counteracting those feelings is to get their girlfriends pregnant. If the girlfriend is working the boy may understandably feel jealous of her economic independence. The West Indian girl in this situation is often confused and guilty, being pulled in different directions. She wants her economic independence but also she wants to hang on to her boyfriend. She feels angry with him for not getting a job. At the same time she knows it is difficult for him to do so. Caught in this tangled web the responsibility for making decisions and persevering with contraception may be too demanding and so fate is allowed to take a hand and pregnancy results. The decision is made for her.

Thus teenage pregnancy may be in response to poor economic prospects and perhaps should be seen as a kind of adaptation, the baby being seen as the passport to independence and a flat. This is often when the help of the social services is sought. The idea of the young West Indian couple working and saving for a home and then having children is in some cases untenable, given the high unemployment, particularly among the younger men. Failure to do well in school may lead to rejection by the parents. This, together with feelings of alienation from white society, has led to the development of a teenage sub-culture where the young people seek emotional and social support from each other. The girls, once they have one child, are in the position of the unmarried mothers discussed earlier but in some ways are more vulnerable. If the baby's father leaves her and she forms a new relationship she may feel that she must have a baby for the new partner in order that he will stay and take care of the other child. Should this relationship break down she is left with two children and so, in extreme cases, it may go on. The more children she has the less the chance of getting married. The girls are often well aware of this and many are making strong attempts to avoid this situation.

Despite the concern with fertility and virility (very few West Indian men referred to the Haringey Domiciliary Service have requested vasectomy) and the anxieties and myths about the contraceptive methods, mentioned earlier in the chapter on methods, there is an interest in family planning and acceptance of it. Many West Indian women, particularly single women, have referred themselves via friends to the Haringey domiciliary service for advice. Those who are already clients of the clinic or domiciliary service constantly refer their friends. Mothers are also now requesting help from the clinic or domiciliary service to come and talk to their daughters about sex to prevent them getting pregnant in their early teens. As the domiciliary FP service in Haringey is in touch with literally hundreds of single mothers it was able to contribute to starting up mothers' groups, particularly for West Indian mothers and their children. Many of the mothers are bored and lonely and the children do not have proper play facilities. Support with family planning has enabled many young mothers to exert more control over their lives and future. (Of the 1725 cases referred to the Haringey DFP Service by health visitors, social workers and self-referred, during 1968-78, 641 (37 per cent) were West Indian or of West Indian origin; of these, 255 (40 per cent) were married and 386 (60 per cent) were single.) (See p. 215 for contrasting features found between the single mother of West Indian origin compared with others referred to the Domiciliary Service.)

SUMMARY: HOW CULTURAL ATTITUDES INFLUENCE CHOICE OF METHOD

Clinical experience indicates that certain methods seem to be followed more often than others by each culture. This seems to depend, in part, on which marital partner is regarded as dominant. Thus in the more patriarchal cultures the husband may either take control of contraception himself or decide what his wife will use. The method chosen is also related to sexual attitudes, particularly to female sexuality. Although somewhat stereotyped attitudes have been presented here from each culture, obviously not all individuals or couples of that culture will conform to them and attitudes are constantly changing.

Attitudes are also influenced by social class and level of education, so that the upper social class and more educated members of each culture will be more flexible in their choice of method.

Cartwright (1976) found that those mothers from India or Pakistan and from Africa or the West Indies were less likely than those born in England, Wales or Scotland to be taking the pill (see table 5). Catholic and Moslem religions were likely to contribute to higher family size as was the lower status of occupations of those from India and Pakistan. Those born in

Table 4: Choice of Method by Ethnic Origin (Haringey Domiciliary Service 1968–1976)

MARRIED

	English/Scots Welsh	Eire	West Indian	Turkish Cypriot	Greek Cypriot	Indian/Pakistani	TOTAL Users
Pill	122 (33%)	29 (24%)	50 (22%)	11 (44%)	7 (13%)	9 (21%)	228 (27%)
Coil	43 (11%)	37 (30%)	36 (16%)	4 (16%)	19 (36%)	18 (43%)	157 (19%)
Sheath	38 (10%)	23 (19%)	47 (21%)	8 (32%)	20 (38%)	10 (24%)	146 (17%)
Cap	4 (1%)	2 (1%)	4 (2%)		1 (2%)	1 (2%)	12 (1%)
Female Sterilisation	75 (20%)	18 (15%)	79 (35%)	2 (8%)	6 (11%)	2 (5%)	182 (22%)
Male Sterilisation	94 (25%)	14 (11%)	9 (4%)	—	—	2 (5%)	119 (14%)
	376=100%	123=100%	225=100%	25=100%	53=100%	42=100%	844=100%

SINGLE

	English/Scots Welsh	Eire	West Indian	Turkish Cypriot	Greek Cypriot	Indian/Pakistani	TOTAL Users
Pill	86 (83%)	5 (45%)	155 (67%)	—	2 (100%)	2 (67%)	250 (72%)
Coil	14 (14%)	6 (55%)	69 (30%)	—	—	1 (43%)	90 (26%)
Sheath	3 (3%)	—	6 (3%)	—	—	—	9 (2%)
	103=100%	11=100%	230=100%	—	22=100%	3=100%	349=100%

(These figures relate to women or couples who had settled on a method. 51 single mothers and 228 married had either not settled on a method, or had moved away, or were pregnant.)

Table 5: Family size at time of interview and place of birth

Married mother's place of birth	England & Wales	Scotland	Ireland	India/Pakistan	West Indies/Africa	Elsewhere
Average no. of children at time of interview	1.90	2.31	2.04	2.51	2.92	1.92
Intended no. of children per woman	2.52	2.74	2.73	3.28	3.43	2.64
Place of birth and current use of contraception						
Female sterilisation	4%	11%	15%	2%	12%	–%
Male sterilisation	4	3	2	2	4	–
Pill	44	45	34	26	25	40
Cap	2	3	–	–	4	–
IUD	5	9	6	5	17	4
Sheath	23	11	11	21	17	14
Coitus interruptus	6	3	6	7	–	10
Safe period	1 ⎫	3 ⎫	4 ⎫	2 ⎫	– ⎫	2 ⎫
Other	2 ⎬ 18%	3 ⎬ 18%	– ⎬ 32%	2 ⎬ 44%	4 ⎬ 21%	6 ⎬ 42%
None	9 ⎭	9 ⎭	22 ⎭	33 ⎭	17 ⎭	24 ⎭
Total no. of cases	1256	36	47	57	25	51

Source: Cartwright, A. *How Many Children?* (Routledge, 1976), Table 95 & Table 96.

the West Indies, Africa, India, Pakistan and Ireland tended to come from large families themselves.

Asian couples Withdrawal and sheath are used to a certain extent prior to professional advice. Reliance is also placed on prolonged lactation. After professional advice all methods may be tried, though vasectomy is not popular.

Cypriot couples Withdrawal and sheath are the predominant methods before and after professional advice. Cypriot women (Greek and Turkish), the older ones particularly, may try the pill and coil, but the couple usually revert to the sheath. Younger women are turning to the pill. Vasectomy will not even be considered as Cypriot men are fearful of its effect on their virility.

Irish couples Initially reliance may be placed on a mixture of abstinence/safe period and withdrawal. Where these methods fail in very fertile couples professional advice may be sought and then the pill and coil are the most favoured. Irish women are reluctant to use the cap. Vasectomy is not too popular. Very fertile women may ask for sterilisation. Cartwright (1976) in her small sample of women born outside the United Kingdom found that a comparatively high proportion of mothers from Ireland were sterilised. (See table on page 244.)

West Indian couples The choice here is influenced by the age group and marital status. The older married couples will use the pill, coil, sheath or cap. West Indian women find the cap an acceptable method and do not have reservations or inhibitions about touching their own genital organs. The older fertile women may seek sterilisation. Vasectomy is not very acceptable. The young West Indian couples tend to rely on withdrawal prior to professional advice. The sheath is not popular. After professional advice reliance is placed on the pill and coil.

An investigation is in progress (FPA/IPPF) to look at attitudes of the different ethnic groups to family planning services. Experience in Haringey with the domiciliary family planning service suggests that this is an acceptable agency for family planning advice where women are too embarrassed and modest to attend a clinic or GP.

PART 3
Abortion

15
Abortion

The Lane Report (1974) stated that, according to the evidence before it, social workers feel that they have so far had little or no training or preparation for dealing with problems related to abortion. Abortion is an emotive subject and one in which the subjective attitudes of the counsellor, doctor or social worker often override the best interests of the women presenting for abortion. It is, perhaps, unfortunate that in a civilised country abortion should still be needed, especially as contraception is now widely and freely available. However, despite this, there will probably always be a need, not just for strictly medical reasons, since methods of contraception fail, couples fail to use contraception conscientiously, and sex, being often unpremeditated, may be unprotected. Also, the circumstances surrounding a planned and wanted pregnancy may change, making it an unwanted one.

HISTORY: ABORTION AND RELIGION

Abortion has been practised throughout history, despite the opposition of the great religions, Hinduism, Buddhism, Judaism and Christianity. It was common in Graeco-Roman times when a variety of drugs and instruments were used. Hippocrates, the father of medicine, advocated violent exercises. (There are women today who believe this to be efficacious.) Early Christianity forbade abortion. However, St Augustine in about the fifth century declared that the embryo *before* quickening did not have a soul and its destruction was punishable by a fine, whereas the quickened embryo had a soul and its destruction was therefore murder. The time of quickening was reckoned to be at forty days. This belief continued until the sixteenth century when the church changed its mind and abortion at any stage was considered murder. At the end of the sixteenth century a return was made to the former judgement, which remained in force until 1869, when the Pope said that the foetus had a soul at conception. In 1930 Pope Pius XI decreed that the life of the unborn child is as sacred as that of the mother and that abortion violates the law of God and nature. This was re-affirmed in the 1968 papal encyclical *Humanae Vitae* which also proclaimed the danger of population control being abused by governments and condemned all interference with the generative process for the purpose of preventing procreation as a crime against God and nature.

The Protestant faith will allow abortion where the mother's life is in danger. Jewish teaching nowadays allows abortion provided there is a consensus of trained opinion after due investigation. The Greek Orthodox and Moslem religions are still opposed to abortion.

ABORTION AND THE LAW

Abortion performed after quickening was judged in England to be a misdemeanour under common law until the early nineteenth century, unless it resulted in the death of the mother, in which case it was a felony and punishable as for murder. Before quickening it was not punishable at all. In 1837 abortion at any time became punishable by transportation or imprisonment. The Offences Against the Person Act of 1861 (which is still in force) made it a felony for a woman to administer a poison to herself, or use an instrument to procure a miscarriage or for anyone else to do so. Nevertheless, nothing was said in the Act to indicate whether abortion in any circumstances might be lawful. The Infant Life (Preservation) Act 1929 provides that it shall be a defence that the act causing the death of the child was done for the purpose only of preserving the life of the mother; thus the discrepancy between these two Acts raised the question as to whether there were any circumstances under the 1861 Act in which a miscarriage might *lawfully* be procured. In 1938 a famous case, *R.* v. *Bourne*, resulted in a liberal interpretation being given to the 1861 and 1929 Acts. Mr Aleck Bourne, a gynaecologist, invited prosecution after terminating the pregnancy of a fourteen-year-old girl, who had been criminally assaulted by a number of soldiers of the Household Cavalry, and was acquitted. His defence was that he had not acted *unlawfully*, and thus this interpretation remained until the 1967 Abortion Act. This new Act was considered necessary because of the imprecise nature of the existing law and hence the risk of prosecution that faced any doctor doing an abortion.

The 1967 Abortion Act

This permits abortion under the following circumstances:

1. The continuance of the pregnancy would induce risk to the life of the pregnant woman greater than if the pregnancy were terminated.

2. The continuance of the pregnancy would involve risk of injury to the physical or mental health of the woman greater than if the pregnancy were terminated.

3. The continuance of the pregnancy would involve risk of injury to the physical or mental health of the existing child(ren) of the family of the pregnant woman greater than if the pregnancy were terminated.

4. There is a substantial risk that if the child were born it would suffer from such physical or mental abnormality as to be seriously handicapped.

The most common grounds for all terminations are grounds 2 and 3. Two doctors are required by law to sign the abortion certificate 'A'. This is usually the general practitioner and the gynaecologist. Before the 1967 Act there was no statutory requirement of notification of abortion, so that precise figures cannot be given. A number of induced abortion cases were recorded but disguised as 'spontaneous abortion' or dilatation and curettage (D&C). Estimates of illegal abortions prior to the Act varied from 111,000–150,000 (Birkett Committee 1939) to 20,000 (Goodhart 1972). It is highly probable that a large number of illegal abortions have been in the past classified either as 'spontaneous' or as 'not specified as induced or spontaneous' rather than placed in the specific illegal category. However, the number of septic abortions (sepsis being a common concomitant of illegal abortions) has declined since 1969. Abortion of all types — spontaneous (a high proportion of all pregnancies end in spontaneous abortion), septic and induced (that is termination of pregnancy) — has always formed a substantial part of the gynaecological work load of the NHS accounting for about one-fifth of all cases in 1959.

Table 6: All Legal Abortions, England & Wales, 1968–77

Source: Registrar General's Statistical Review for England and Wales 1969–73, Supplement on Abortion. (OPCS Monitor Ref. AB 76/7, AB 77/2, AB 77/1, AB 78/10.

	TOTAL Residents and Non-Residents	Abortions Under 20 Residents	Abortions Under 16 Residents	Nos of Non-Residents*
1968	23,641	4,008	543	1,300
1969	54,819	10,166	1,174	4,990
1970	86,565	15,955	1,732	10,603
1971	126,777	20,500	2,296	32,207
1972	159,884	24,600	2,804	51,319
1973	167,149	26,590	3,090	56,581
1974	163,117	27,540	3,335	53,672
1975	140,251	27,670	3,570	34,027
1976	128,813	27,388	3,425	26,901
1977	132,999	28,215	3,624	30,762

*Non-Residents include women from Scotland, N. Ireland, Channel Islands, Eire, Europe and other countries.
Less than 1 per cent of women from foreign countries had their abortions through the NHS.

Abortions by Marital Status of England & Wales Residents, 1969–76

	All	Single	Married	Other (widows, divorced, separated)
1969	49,829	22,287	22,979	4,563
1970	75,962	34,492	34,314	7,156
1971	94,570	44,302	41,536	8,732
1972	108,565	51,115	46,894	10,556
1973	110,568	52,899	46,766	10,903
1974	109,445	53,321	45,102	11,022
1975	106,224	52,335	43,066	10,823
1976	101,912	50,901	40,311	10,700

50 per cent of all women who had an abortion had had a previous birth, stillbirth or miscarriage. The highest proportion of both single and married women was between 20 and 34 years. The majority of abortions occurring under 20 are to single women.

DIAGNOSIS OF PREGNANCY

By the woman

Pregnancy may be suspected by missed periods in a woman whose periods are regular. Breasts become fuller and tender and urine is passed more frequently. She may also have morning sickness.

By the doctor

1. From the history: menstrual history and symptoms.
2. Examination: vaginal examination. The uterus starts to enlarge at about 6 to 8 weeks of pregnancy. Breasts may be slightly enlarged, the pigmentation of the nipple area may be darker and the veins more prominent on the breast.
3. Pregnancy tests: these are immunological tests using a drop of urine. These tests become positive indicating that a woman is pregnant *two weeks* after a missed period, i.e. when the woman is *six weeks* pregnant, because pregnancy is dated from the first day of the last menstrual period. There are two tests: the latex test, which takes two minutes to get a result and the haemagglutination test, which takes two hours. The tests are reliable when performed by a person who is familiar with the technique and should be performed with controlled tests. These tests ideally should be done in a clinic or by the hospital or GP who has the woman's history and has examined her, rather than the local chemist, because of false negatives. A false negative can occur if the test is done too early. It should, therefore, be repeated one to two weeks later. False negatives can occur in menopausal women. Home testing kits are not reliable.

THE UNWANTED PREGNANCY

What a woman does when she suspects she is pregnant and does not want it can vary enormously. The more knowledgeable articulate woman, provided she is not ambivalent about the pregnancy, tends to go sooner to the GP or clinic for help. The woman who is not so well informed (usually of a lower socio-economic group) may either deny the pregnancy ('I am not really pregnant — the blood is blocked up') and not see a doctor until two or three periods are missed, by which time she is 10—12 weeks pregnant; or she may try home-made remedies to 'bring on' the period, such as hot baths, alcohol, purgatives and so on. When she does go to her doctor she may request tablets to 'bring on' her period. It is unfortunate that many GPs used to prescribe a hormone preparation to cause withdrawal bleeding. They have now been advised by the Committee on the Safety of Medicines against this, as there is a possibility that they may lead to foetal abnormalities. By the time a woman is finally convinced that she is pregnant and seeks an abortion she may well be 12 to 14 weeks pregnant. A hospital appointment may not be available for two to three weeks so she may be 16 weeks before she has an abortion. Abortions done at this time are more dangerous. The Lane Report showed that single women consult their doctor later than married women.

When a woman requests an abortion the ease with which she will obtain one depends on a number of factors:

a) how far the pregnancy has advanced — the earlier it is performed the better it is for the woman's health;

b) the attitude of the GP or clinic;

c) the attitude of the local gynaecologist.

There are considerable regional variations. In Newcastle and Aberdeen 96 per cent of women get NHS abortions, in Wolverhampton only 7 per cent, in Birmingham 10 per cent and in Coventry 16 per cent (Lane Report 1974).

Abortions are performed through the following agencies:

1. NHS gynaecological departments, with variations as shown above.

2. Private bed — costing several hundred pounds. The private sector was used before 1967 by social classes I and II. A turnover of £3 million per year in Harley Street is quoted (Peel & Potts 1969, p. 27).

3. Private nursing homes, which are linked to the Pregnancy Advisory Services, which are charitable non-profit-making.

PREGNANCY ADVISORY SERVICES

The 1967 Abortion Act was permissive, not mandatory, and gave consultants great freedom. In Birmingham 5.6 per cent of its gynaecological beds (it has 948) were used for notified abortions under the Act compared to 10.3 per cent in

Newcastle (which has 798 beds) (Lane Report 1974). Because of these geographical inequalities two registered charities, the British Pregnancy Advisory Service, which has clinics in Birmingham, Brighton, Coventry, Leeds and Liverpool, and the Pregnancy Advisory Service, based in London, were set up to meet local needs. The cost is about £77.00, which is reduced in needy cases. The woman can refer herself, or be referred by her GP or the family planning clinic. She is seen by a social worker, who takes her social history and counsels the woman, discussing all the alternatives to an abortion, and then by a doctor who examines her and confirms the pregnancy. If the woman has grounds under the Act she is then referred to a gynaecologist. The abortion is done in a nursing home. The Lane Report on the whole praised the services but made three criticisms:

a) they came nearer to performing abortions on demand or on request than Parliament intended;

b) they do not always consult with or even notify the patient's own doctor concerning her abortion;

c) although their charges are moderate compared with those of a commercial profit-making part of the sector they are still enough to enable very high fees to be paid to the doctors employed.

In 1975 about 48 per cent of abortions were done under the NHS, 30 per cent through the Pregnancy Advisory Services and 22 per cent through the private sector. In 1976, 49,837 women in England and Wales had NHS abortions compared to 51,166 in the charitable and private sectors.

The Lane Report represents a careful and thorough look at the working of the 1967 Abortion Act. It recommended that doctors should continue to make the decision about abortions, that abortion work should not be restricted to the NHS and that the wording of the Act laying down criteria for abortions should be left unamended. It also recommended an upper time limit for abortions of 24 weeks. At present it is 28 weeks. Less than 1 per cent of abortions are done after 20 weeks.

The majority of doctors have expressed themselves satisfied with the working of the 1967 Act.

METHODS OF PERFORMING AN ABORTION

The method used varies with the duration of the pregnancy and whether the woman has had previous pregnancies.

Methods for early abortions, up to 12 weeks

Suction method

A plastic tube or cannula attached to a suction pump sucks out the contents of the uterus through the vagina. This is the most commonly used method of performing early abortions. It is quick (5–10 minutes), safe (provided there are no medical or gynaecological complications), and cheap. Blood loss is minimal.

It can be used to perform *outpatient abortions* (the so-called day-care abortions) using local anaesthetic up to 10 weeks pregnancy with no or minimal stretching of the neck of the womb. If local anaesthetic is used, the patient must be informed and cooperative. In those hospitals where this is done the social worker who has counselled the woman prior to the operation and explained it to her stays with her throughout the procedure. About 12 per cent of women (12,000) have day-care abortions, half in the NHS and half through the Pregnancy Advisory Services. Unfortunately, day-care facilities are not available in all NHS hospitals and so some women having early abortions have to stay one or two nights in hospital. For 10–12 weeks pregnancy the suction method can also be used but under a *general anaesthetic* in women who have not been pregnant previously. In those women who have had previous pregnancies this method can be used until 14 weeks.

Dilatation and curettage (D&C)

This method was commonly used before the suction method became available. It is performed under a general anaesthetic and the woman stays one or two nights in hospital. The neck of the womb is stretched (dilated) and the contents of the womb are scraped out (curettage). It is not as safe as the suction method and there is greater risk of damaging the cervix so that the woman may miscarry with subsequent pregnancies. Blood loss tends to be greater with D&C.

Methods for late abortions, 14–24 weeks

Late abortions are much more dangerous and unpleasant for the woman and require a longer hospital stay, approximately 3 days.

Non-surgical method

The uterus is injected with a urea solution after some of the fluid surrounding the foetus has been removed. This results in foetal death. Prostaglandin is then injected into the uterus; this causes the woman to go into labour and to expel the dead foetus. Pain is usually relieved by epidural anaesthetic. This method is used from the 16th to the 24th week. There is a risk of perforating the bladder if this is done earlier. Afterwards a brief curettage under general anaesthetic is given to ensure that the uterus is empty. Should any after-birth remain it can lead to severe haemorrhage.

Surgical methods

These are rarely used now as they are associated with high mortality rates. *Hysterotomy* is a mini-caesarean. It can be combined with sterilisation. The woman has to be in hospital for eight days. *Hysterectomy* involves removal of the uterus and is only done where there is a serious abnormality of the uterus or cervix.

Criminal abortion

The techniques vary for this and each culture seems to have its own patent remedy or remedies. The most popular method is a syringe filled with soapy solution or Dettol. Knitting needles have been used together with a wide variety of pills which contain ergot, quinine and other chemicals that can poison or kill the pregnant woman or produce a grossly abnormal baby. The dangers of criminal abortion are haemorrhage, air or fluid embolism which can lead to paralysis or death, and infection that can be severe enough to cause death. In 1963, 239 women died from delivery and the complications of childbirth, 49 died from abortion — spontaneous and criminal. The Lane Committee found that the number of prosecutions under the Offences Against the Person Act 1861 had fallen since the 1967 Abortion Act. The majority of senior police officers consider that the number of illegal abortions has decreased since the 1967 Act, though the Lane Committee felt it was unlikely to disappear because of the ease and convenience of self-induced or back-street abortion, despite its being more dangerous. In 1974 there were 370 cases treated in hospital where the main diagnosis was illegal abortion and 540 discharges from hospital of patients with septic (and therefore likely to be illegal) abortion (Hansard 1978(1).

Figure 3: Total deaths due to abortion, all causes, England & Wales, 1928—1970

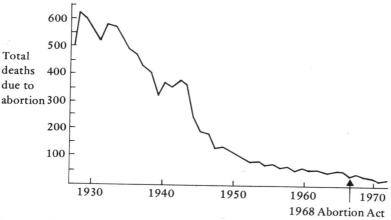

1968 Abortion Act

Source: Potts, Diggory & Peel, *Abortion*. Cambridge University Press.

Table 7: Total Number of Legal Abortions during 1968—1973 and death rate per 100,000 abortions, England & Wales, by length of pregnancy: Residents

Length of pregnancy	Nos aborted 1968—1973	Death rate per 100,000 abortions
Under 9 weeks	80,847	5
9—12 weeks	269,168	9.7
13—16 weeks	89,985	24
17 weeks and over	21,826	73

Source: Huntingford, P. *Abortion* NHS and the Charities Birth Control Trust, 1977.

EFFECTS OF ABORTION

Mortality

Fatality is highest following hysterectomy, hysterotomy and non-surgical methods and of abortion that is combined with sterilisation and lowest with dilatation and curettage and similar techniques. This explains the need to perform abortions as early as possible.

In 1974 death from D&C or suction in all age groups of abortions done in 12 weeks or under was 3 to 4 per 100,000 abortions. Maternal mortality excluding abortion was 13 per 100,000. It is safer to have an abortion in the first three months of pregnancy than to have the child. What is perhaps more disturbing is that according to the latest figures on abortion it is *safer* to have an abortion *outside* the NHS. Brewer (1978) commented that a woman was seven times more likely to die if she has her abortion through the NHS. This was based on the answer to a Parliamentary Question (Hansard 978[2]) that the death rate per 100,000 abortions was 1.84 outside the NHS (that is through Pregnancy Advisory Services and private), but 6.8 within the NHS.

 Possible explanations for this are that a higher proportion of late abortions are done within the NHS compared to the private sector; cases where there are medical or gynaecological complications are more likely to be seen under the NHS; and poorer and thus less healthy women are more likely to have abortions through the NHS.

Morbidity

Physical effects of abortion

Haemorrhage Very rarely is this enough to require blood transfusion. With the suction method blood loss is minimal.

Infection This may vary from slight to severe. If severe it may lead to infection of the fallopian tubes and subsequent sterility. There is little statistical evidence on this (though it was a common occurrence after criminal abortion). It is not clear whether the risk of pelvic infection is more or less after therapeutic abortion than after childbirth (Lane Report 1974).

Damage to the uterus and/or tearing of the cervix. This is more likely to occur when the neck of the womb has been stretched or dilated. This can lead subsequently to spontaneous abortion or premature labour. Reports about this have come mainly from East Europe though, as the Lane Report pointed out, there is little reliable controlled data available. Thus, in order to assess these risks prospective and carefully planned studies are required comparing the long-term results of induced abortions with those in suitable control cases of women in early pregnancy matched for age parity, social class, and obstetric history wishing to continue their pregnancy. Damage to the uterus (perforations) is rare (3—4 cases per 1,000).

Operative techniques carry the risk of developing thrombosis which may be fatal.

It must be borne in mind that the alternative to abortion is childbirth, and infection, haemorrhage, thrombosis and reduced fertility can and do occur with it. Hence once pregnancy has occurred these problems cannot be avoided.

Psychological effects of abortion

One of the major difficulties in trying to assess the psychological effects of abortion lies in dissociating the effects of the operation from the circumstances surrounding the pregnancy itself and why it is unwanted. Much also depends on how difficult it is to obtain an abortion and how the woman is treated by those who care for her during the abortion. An additional factor is that women seeking an abortion often feel guilty about doing so and in consequence are extremely sensitive to professional attitudes and may over-react to them.

The Marriage Guidance Council in a memorandum to the Lane Committee stated that many of the clients who come to them are troubled by past events such as abortion. But how far is this due to the client anxiously seeking for some past cause to blame for the present state of distress? People who are depressed often feel that they are being punished for past misdeeds and an abortion may be seen in this context, especially where it had to be hidden from relatives or partner. It must be remembered that not only was it more difficult to obtain an abortion in the past but also there were fewer opportunities for the woman to talk about her feelings in relation to the abortion.

The Lane Report found that the risk of serious mental illness after a therapeutic abortion was slight, occurring in about 2 per cent of cases. Therapeutic abortion appeared to have little influence on the course of an existing mental illness such as schizophrenia. Emotional stress is more likely in late abortions, as these are like miniature labours and the distress suffered by the nurses present may communicate itself to the woman. The Lane Report (1974) concluded that significant psychiatric sequelae of abortion (and of refusal of abortion) are more likely in those who have been temperamentally unstable prior to the pregnancy. In a wide review of the literature between 1934 and 1965 dealing with the psychiatric sequelae of abortion, Simon & Senturia (1966) found that the incidence of severe guilt was reported as between zero and 43 per cent! The Osofskys (1974) reviewing the literature concluded that personal conviction often outweighed the evidence since the conclusions of different authors ranged from the view that psychiatric illness almost always occurred after therapeutic abortion to the view that it was virtually absent in most cases. There was also a frequent failure to study the pre-abortion psychological state. Studies could also be biased if one of the conditions for obtaining abortion was psychological illness.

The Osofskys also concluded that as there are some 4,000 documented postpartum psychoses requiring hospitalisation in the United States per year (about 1 to 2 per 1,000 deliveries) there should also be a sizeable number of women hospitalised for post-abortion psychoses if abortion was as traumatic as term delivery. There is hardly any mention of post-abortion psychosis in the literature. The Osofskys make the further observation that no study has yet been able to predict precisely which women will react adversely to pregnancy or to termination.

Tietze & Lewit (1972) in a follow-up of 73,000 legally aborted women found that the incidence of major psychiatric complications (virtually synonymous with admission to a psychiatric ward) was 0.2 − 0.4 per 1,000 abortions. However, it should be noted that diagnostic concepts differ from those used in Britain and the follow-up period was short. Brewer (1977 [1]) reported an incidence of post-abortion psychosis of 0.3 per 1,000 legal abortions compared to an incidence of puerperal psychosis (that is after birth) of 1.7 per 1,000 deliveries. (Brewer's figures were obtained from twenty consultant psychiatrists who were asked to record all patients admitted under their care who had had a legal abortion during the previous three months over a fifteen-month period. The consultants served a catchment area population of 1,333,000.) Greer *et al.* (1976) followed up 360 single and married women who underwent termination in the first three months of pregnancy. Each patient received brief counselling before the operation. Follow-up examinations were carried out by means of detailed Structured Interviews at three months and between fifteen and twenty-four months. Outcome was assessed in terms of psychiatric symptoms, guilt feelings and adjustment in marital and other interpersonal relationships, sexual responsiveness and work record. The results showed that significant improvement had occurred at follow-up in all areas save marital adjustment where there was no significant change. Adverse psychiatric and social sequelae were rare.

One way of assessing the extent of guilty feelings and the pressure to relieve them after abortion is to see how soon afterwards the woman becomes pregnant again, since this is usually a form of expiation. Few studies have looked at this with the notable exception of Ekblad (1955). Whereas he found that only 1 per cent of 479 women legally aborted in Sweden on psychiatric grounds had had a major psychiatric disability following the abortion, 40 per cent of the married women had become pregnant within twenty-two months of the abortion, the majority being unintentional. Of the unmarried women under twenty-six years, 10 per cent had become pregnant by another man unintentionally within six months, 18 per cent by one year and 25 per cent by two years. Only 10 per cent had become intentionally pregnant within two years. These findings would appear to suggest that some of these women were ambivalent about the original pregnancy and were possibly under pressure (from relatives, partners, doctors) to have an abortion. They would also appear to indicate a need for careful counselling. From clinical experience it seems that while most women having an abortion do suffer from transient depression and feelings of regret and guilt (made worse if the woman is treated unkindly), nevertheless these feelings are usually outweighed by an almost overwhelming sense of relief.

EFFECTS OF REFUSAL OF ABORTION

The mother

It is not possible to determine how many women who seek abortion are refused. A number who are, will obtain an abortion either at another hospital or privately or illegally. Some women who are refused feel relieved, possibly because they have been given 'permission' to have a baby. This may occur where pressure has been put on them by partner/parent to have an abortion. There has been little research into the psychological effects in women refused abortion. Hook (1963) found that a quarter of 249 women who were refused abortion seen 7—11 years later had adjusted poorly to the refusal. One-third of the women studied by Pare & Raven (1970) who were refused abortion, regretted that termination had not been carried out and many admitted to feelings of resentment towards the child.

The child

Some women happily accept the child if abortion is refused — in some cases, as stated earlier, glad to be given 'permission' to have the baby — but others do not. What happens to the child in these circumstances? There are two longitudinal studies done on the fate of the children of unwanted pregnancies. The earliest is that made by Forssman & Thuwe (1966) in Sweden who followed up 120 children for twenty-one years whose mothers had been refused abortion. These were compared with an appropriate control series. At the time these women requested abortion this was not allowed on socio-medical grounds (that is, where the birth and care of the expected child will seriously undermine the woman's mental or physical health). The unwanted children were born to mothers whose average age was thirty years. The control group mothers were aged twenty-eight. 26 per cent of the unwanted children were born out of wedlock against only 7 per cent of the control group, though they were of comparable social groups. Eight of the unwanted children were adopted by others not their real parents (seven of these children were illegitimate). Data were collected from civil and ecclesiastical registry offices, social agencies, school and military authorities and all the psychiatric in-patient and out-patient departments wherever the subject had lived. The study revealed that 60 per cent of the unwanted children had an insecure background as against 28 per cent of the control group, as measured by the child being placed in a foster home or children's home and parents being divorced before the child was fifteen years old. The unwanted children were more often registered for antisocial and criminal behaviour. They got public assistance more often. The girls married earlier and had children earlier than the control series. The authors conclude that the very fact that a woman seeks an authorised abortion, no matter how trivial the grounds may appear to others, means that the expected child will run a larger risk than its peers of 'an inferior standing in life'. It was their opinion that the legislation on therapeutic termination of pregnancy should also consider the social risks to which the expected child will be exposed.

A legitimate criticism of this study is that since 26 per cent of the unwanted children were born out of wedlock it is possible that this alone could have accounted for the findings. The authors do not state whether the above features occurred more among the illegitimate than the legitimate children. Nevertheless, the fact remains that unwanted children in this study were born into a worse situation than other children and provides evidence (1) that the unwanted child may have to face greater disadvantages physically and mentally than a wanted one and (2) of the necessity of taking social factors into account when women seek abortions.

The second later study was carried out in Czechoslovakia by Dytrych *et al.* (1975). It is based on 233 children born to mothers who had been refused legal abortion in Czechoslovakia in the years 1961–63. A control group of children was matched for sex, birth order, number of siblings, marital status of mother and occupation of father. The two groups were compared in over 400 different ways. Only slight differences were shown between the two groups apart from language proficiency, which was significantly poorer in the study group. The author concluded that the belief that a child unwanted during pregnancy remains unwanted is not necessarily true. However, the opposite notion, that the birth of a child brings a complete change in attitude and that every woman who becomes a mother will love her child, is also untrue. The child of a mother denied an abortion is born in a potentially handicapped situation. It must be noted that this study was based on a small number of women refused an abortion out of 25,000 who were granted an abortion. It may have been that those women who were refused were ambivalent about an abortion anyway.

ABORTION COUNSELLING

Much concern was expressed in the Lane Report on the need for adequate counselling facilities for women seeking abortion and that counselling should provide opportunities for discussion, information, explanation and advice. Those women who go to the British Pregnancy Advisory Service and the London Pregnancy Advisory Service do receive counselling. However, within the NHS there is enormous variation. In some hospitals every woman requesting termination is seen by a social worker who in some cases, as stated earlier, sees the woman through the abortion if this is done under local anaesthetic as an out-patient procedure. In others only women who have been refused abortion are seen by a social worker. According to the Lane Report, most hospitals seem to have a mixed approach but some emphasise one direction more than another depending on the hospital's policy on abortion. If the policy is very 'liberal' or 'illiberal' then social circumstances might play very little part in determining the decision about abortion and thus the social work service tends to be client-orientated. In the first situation this involves dealing with underlying problems of providing support while the patient is in hospital. In the second, the social workers are more likely to be involved in dealing with the consequences of refusal. Where abortion is performed on a more selective basis the social worker might be asked to obtain a social report to help the consultant make a decision; more rarely social workers are asked to help the patient reach a decision or to provide help when underlying problems have been perceived by the doctor. Social workers are not involved for very long and, therefore, there are very few long-term follow-ups except in the case of a refusal. The age and marital status of the women referred vary, some hospitals sending all young and single to social workers, others, the older married women. There are no accurate figures on the number of women who are seen by a social worker prior to the abortion and estimates of between 0.6 per cent and 32 per cent have been given (Lane Report 1974) with enormous regional variations.

What is abortion counselling?

Simms (1974) suggests that there are basically two kinds of abortion counselling:

a) the simpler kind of offering information about the law, the abortion procedure, birth control, housing, etc.;

b) the more complex kind which is psychiatric or psycho-sexual and is probably needed by only a small minority of women.

Counselling is a term which can be used imprecisely and so widely as to be almost meaningless. Thus it is often thought to be synonymous with advice and information-giving, as in Simms's simpler kind of counselling. However, counselling really refers to an exploration and clarification of feelings and motivations and also the identification of conflict and ambivalence. The counsellor acts as a kind of catalyst, enabling the person to understand himself and to make decisions in the light of this new understanding. Cheetham (1977) explores counselling and the unwanted pregnancy although abortion counselling itself is dealt with in the final chapter.

Do all women need counselling?

Abortion itself can be seen as an 'acute psychiatric emergency' (Leiter 1972) or as a more commonplace event. Those holding the latter view argue that as women have always had abortions in the past (and illegal ones, at that) without much emotional damage it is unnecessary to make too much fuss. Information together with back-up psychiatric facilities, should they be necessary, is all that is needed. What do women themselves want? A recent study carried out in Denmark (IPP 1974) of women attending a Mothers' Aid Centre requesting abortion showed that only 1 per cent availed themselves of the offer of counselling after information about the abortion procedure and alternatives to it had been discussed. It is unknown what proportion of women need counselling. The problem and indeed the skill lies in identifying those who do. *Should* all women requesting abortion receive counselling? Certainly those women who are ambivalent about pregnancy need to be identified and counselled. There is a danger, however, that counselling could be seen as, or indeed made, an additional hurdle to be overcome in order to achieve an abortion. The woman will then be compliant to gain her end. Indeed, it could be argued that when the woman knows that she does not have to convince any professional person, be it doctor, nurse, social worker or counsellor, of the legitimacy and sincerity of her request, the truth will be reached that much sooner. The time factor imposes constraints on the decision about abortion, since a decision has to be made quickly, often in a matter of a day or 1–2 weeks at the most. This can be frustrating for the counsellor or social worker who may feel that the woman has not explained her situation fully and that a decision is being taken at a time when the woman is in a highly emotional state and which could change if more time were available. There is some uncertainty as to who should counsel women for abortion. Simms (1974) recommends in her report lay counsellors with the right personal outlook and attributes and with suitable in-service training programmes, since there are not (and not likely to be) enough qualified social workers. The Standing Conference for the Advancement of Counselling, now the British Association for Counselling (BAC), rejected the idea of the wholesale interposition of lay or of specialist abortion counsellors. It urged the encouragement of more skilful and sympathetic attitudes within the existing helping professions. This would seem essential, particularly in the case of the medical profession. A study of abortion in Aberdeen (Horobin 1973) showed that Aberdeen doctors were in many subtle ways socially and morally selective in their abortion decisions. Thus the decision whether to abort involved 'moral judgements and assessments of social deprivation — clearly not within the province of their professional expertise' and intuition — 'thought she would become more depressed', 'thought she was fond of children'. In Sydney, Australia, women who have had abortions help to counsel those requesting abortion at Pre-Term, which is similar in organisation and function to the Pregnancy Advisory Service in England and is also a non-profit-making charitable trust. Some family planning clinics (e.g. Brook) and some AHA clinics do pregnancy testing and offer advice and information and counselling where it is needed. Ideally all family planning clinics should offer this service as complementary to their family planning role.

Case history: loneliness A married woman of thirty with three children referred herself to the domiciliary family planning service through a friend. She was pregnant and requested abortion. Her husband was in prison and as she did not anticipate having sex with anyone she was not using any form of contraception. She was lonely and isolated. A friend had suggested going to a party. She drank too much and had intercourse, though her recollection of this was hazy. She cared about her husband and did not want to put her marriage in jeopardy. She was helped to have an abortion. She decided to take the pill and was followed up by the domiciliary service for a short time and then referred to a family planning clinic.

Abortion counselling and the social worker

The situation regarding abortion counselling facing the social worker in the hospital or family planning clinics is different from that facing the local authority based social worker. The social worker in the former case will know whether the woman is definitely pregnant and how far the pregnancy is advanced, as the woman will have seen a doctor or had a referral letter from a doctor.

However, in the case of the field social worker who may be approached by a woman, usually from a lower socio-economic group, with an unwanted pregnancy, who has not seen a doctor, it will be necessary to refer her to her GP to ascertain the presence and duration of the pregnancy, because she may not be pregnant at all or the pregnancy may be too advanced for an abortion. Where the woman does not for personal reasons wish to see the GP or where she feels he may be inimical to her request, referral to a family planning clinic or a domiciliary family planning service where this is available will be necessary.

For some women such referral without detailed exploration of emotional difficulties may be all that is required. However, for others much more help may be needed — help to make a decision, and because the abortion request may be a cry for help with other problems. In the latter circumstance the women (or girls) may well have tried other means of calling attention to themselves such as taking drugs, drink or getting into trouble with the law. If the abortion only is dealt with, the underlying problems may lead to severe depression and even suicide attempts.

The social worker may already be working with the woman or girl, for example, where the girl is under a supervision order. This places the social worker in the unique situation of being able to give much more comprehensive care than other professionals and to do follow-up work. Thus the social worker is often in the best position to determine which women will need particular care.

One possible view of abortion counselling is that its main, if not sole purpose is to enable the woman to make a decision about whether or not to have an abortion. However, if the abortion experience is to be a learning one for the woman (and couple, where the man is involved) then abortion counselling must encompass more than this.

The aims of abortion counselling

1. To help the woman arrive at a decision where she has not already done so.

2. To provide information about the abortion itself and its alternatives, i.e. having the baby, keeping it or having it adopted and what help the woman can expect if she decides to do this, e.g. with housing, finance, so that the decision is made in the full knowledge of all the possibilities.

3. To help the woman to fully express and cope with her feelings regarding the pregnancy and the abortion both *before* and *after*. The relief experienced after an abortion may be replaced by regret and guilt that it was necessary. For some women the feeling of failure can be very strong after an abortion. Support is needed for these women, particularly for the young.

4. To help the woman understand how and why the pregnancy 'happened' and what aspects of her behaviour led to it. This will serve the dual purpose of enabling her to cope with her feelings about the abortion and take responsibility for it and also, it is hoped, prevent a similar situation occurring.

5. To advise and help with contraception.

In order to achieve these aims the social worker will need to know something of the circumstances preceding and surrounding the pregnancy, the feelings the woman has about herself, the kind of relationships she makes, and her life-style and her attitudes towards sex and contraception. Some of these aspects have already been covered in Part 2, so only the main points will be reiterated here. If the girl or woman is on the social worker's caseload then much of this information will already be known and the main emphasis in counselling may lie in interpreting the behaviour that led to the pregnancy and giving support after the abortion together with contraceptive follow-up.

Before examining the above-mentioned areas in greater detail it is essential that the social worker (or indeed any professional from whom the woman seeks help) should make a simple statement about their attitude towards abortion. If they are opposed to abortion on religious or personal grounds then the woman should be informed of this and referred elsewhere. If there are no ethical objections to abortion then the social worker should make it clear from the outset that he/she is there to help the woman make her decision (if she is uncertain what to do) and to support her in whatever decision she does finally make. Such a statement enables the woman to relax and talk freely and honestly without feeling that she needs to convince the social worker that she needs an abortion. Despite popular belief, the decision to seek or have an abortion is rarely an easy one. Women come with a mixture of feelings and fantasies — guilt and shame about the pregnancy occurring and the need to have an abortion, a sense of failure and a fear of the reaction of professionals. She may believe that she will be punished in some way (unfortunately she may be by some professionals who perhaps hope that by treating the woman like a naughty child she will not repeat the 'misdemeanour'). She may, of course, want to be punished, seeing this as her due for her 'wicked' behaviour, especially when she feels that sexual enjoyment is wrong. Fear and anxiety may be hidden by an outwardly aggressive and hostile attitude demanding her 'rights'. If she fears her request will be met by refusal she may act in an hysterical and desperate way. This is the legacy of having to convince the professional worker that unless an abortion was granted, a breakdown or suicide attempt would be the consequence. Perhaps in no other area of medical care have women been so browbeaten, humiliated and forced to beg, plead and cajole. Thus for all these reasons the social worker needs to make his/her position clear. As stated earlier, abortion is an emotive subject and no one can feel neutral about it. The social worker will need to assess how far his views, whether strongly for or against, interfere with helping the woman and serving her best interests.

Main areas to be explored in abortion counselling

Although the following aspects concerned with abortion counselling are presented separately, for the sake of clarity and to provide a guiding framework, it is not suggested that they should be followed in sequence. As with counselling in other situations, the information gathered will often appear disconnected until it is looked at as a whole.

Circumstances surrounding the pregnancy

The pregnancy may 'happen' when the woman or girl is faced with a difficult or painful choice, e.g. staying on at school, going to'college, finding a job or when there are conflicts with the partner or the family (particularly in the case of teenagers). Thus it may be hoped that the pregnancy will free her from taking responsibility about the choice or will resolve conflicts with the partner or family. However, once the pregnancy has occurred, the reality of coping with a child may be too great and abortion requested.

The circumstances surrounding the pregnancy may be related to the woman's life-style. This may be unstable with frequent job and address changes which may go with a casual approach to relationships and contraception. Loneliness, isolation and separation from the regular sexual partner can have a similar effect. A change in life-style, e.g. leaving home, going to university, sharing a flat with friends, may mean greater freedom for which the girl is not prepared.

Women under stress, e.g. finding their studies or job too exacting, may not be able consciously to admit this to themselves and so may allow a pregnancy to happen.

Relationships

The kind of relationships formed by the woman and their stability are important in several respects. They may provide an indication of the way the woman feels about herself — the poorer her self-esteem, the more casual her relationships. As a general rule, the more casual or unstable the relationship, the greater the risk of an unwanted pregnancy since contraception is unlikely to be used (Lambert 1971).

Pregnancy may be used to test a partner's affection and/or committal, particularly in the young and those involved in an extramarital relationship. Extramarital affairs do not necessarily indicate that the people involved wish to end their marriages (e.g. one of the marital partners may be ill or handicapped prohibiting sexual activity) and a pregnancy could prove disastrous. These cases need to be handled with tact and sensitivity and without moralising. Pregnancy may be used to prevent the break-up of a relationship. The break-up often precedes or takes place at the same time as the abortion request. Battered wives on the point of leaving their husbands are often deliberately made pregnant by their husbands in the hope of preventing this.

The stability of the relationship can affect the use of contraception (see below) and the outcome of the abortion studies done on psychological morbidity indicate that this is worse where the woman's relationships are poor and non-supportive.

Attitudes towards femininity and fertility

The reassurance given by a pregnancy may be needed by women uncertain or anxious about their femininity or fertility, from whatever cause (e.g. doubt as to their sexual attractiveness, negative parental attitudes towards their developing sexuality), though they may not want a child.

Women fearful of childbirth or of the responsibility of motherhood may panic when they learn they are pregnant and seek an abortion. Paradoxically, perhaps, stereotyped feminine attitudes tend to be associated with problems with pregnancy and childbirth (Breen 1975). Doubts about their mothering capacities, possibly due to parental over-emphasis on academic achievement at the expense of other aspects of the personality, may lead some women to seek an abortion when pregnant.

It needs to be stressed that unless the underlying reasons for the doubts and uncertainties connected with femininity and fertility are explored and understood, further unwanted pregnancies may occur.

Attitudes towards contraception and sex

Apart from the fear and embarrassment surrounding sex and contraception which prevent contraceptive advice being sought, it should be remembered that the effective use of contraception is determined by the stability of the relationship. Erratic use and non-use are associated with casual or unstable relationships. Where there is a fear or a need to test committal contraception may also be used haphazardly. Erratic use, especially in someone who was previously an effective user, indicates ambivalence about a possible pregnancy and/or uncertainty about the future. Erratic use occurs in the early stages of a relationship and when it is coming to an end.

Pregnancy may, of course, be the result of a method failure.

Why abortion is being requested

1. It may be the result of a confrontation with reality. It may be realised that a pregnancy will not be a solution to other problems or resolve dilemmas about choice; nor will it prevent the break-up of a relationship, hold a marriage together or force a partner into marriage.

The woman, whether married or single, who already has children, may feel that another child will strain her own or the family's emotional, physical and financial resources. This may occur particularly where there is a large family or a member of the family or the woman herself is handicapped or ill.

If she is single with no children she may feel, particularly if her partner has left her, that it would be unfair to the child to go through with the pregnancy. She may feel she is not ready emotionally and financially for the responsibility of a child, particularly if she is young.

The woman would seem to be the best judge of her circumstances in the above-mentioned situations.

2. Pregnancy may be the result of incest or rape.

3. The request for abortion may be a request for help with other problems — loneliness, inability to sustain relationships, poor self-esteem, doubts about femininity, sexual and marital difficulties, problems with children, growing old.

4. The request may be due to the pressure of others:

a) the partner

   (i) where there is a fear of being forced into marriage.
   (ii) where there has been prior agreement not to have children and then there is a change of mind in one partner.

   Pregnancies are then engineered. Pills are forgotten. Coils are pulled out. Sheaths tear. The other partner feels cheated. The choice may be between continuing with the marriage or the pregnancy.

b) relatives. This tends to occur with the single pregnant teenager whose parents are opposed to the pregnancy. It may also occur with single mentally or physically handicapped girls where the parents may feel that the burden of a child is too great for the girl and for themselves.

c) doctors. The woman may be advised to have an abortion on medical grounds, because of risk to her health or that of the child. This can be particularly disturbing where pregnancy has been planned.

This group can face some of the most difficult problems in abortion counselling. There are no easy solutions. The social worker should attempt to enable the girl or woman to face and own reality while at the same time acknowledging and helping her to cope with the pain and grief this entails. In some cases the social worker will need to assess whether the woman genuinely wants an abortion or whether she is ambivalent despite her request.

As stated earlier, ambivalence can be revealed by the erratic use of contraception. It can also be demonstrated by the woman presenting at a late state in the pregnancy. She may hope that the boyfriend/husband will change his mind and accept the pregnancy or that it will prevent the break-up of the relationship. She may be seeking permission to have the baby against pressure from partner or relatives by being told that it is too late for an abortion.

(Of course there are other reasons for presenting late:

a) the denial of the possibility of pregnancy until it is obvious to others, particularly in the case of teenagers afraid of parental reaction;

b) guilt and shame about becoming pregnant and having a sexual relationship;

c) ignorance about where to go to get help;

d) professionals being unhelpful.)

Ambivalence can also be demonstrated by the woman's choice of agency to help her. Significantly, for example, 90 per cent of the women who go to the Pregnancy Advisory Service actually have the abortion. Of the remaining 10 per cent a few are refused abortion because the pregnancy is too advanced, a few have spontaneous abortions and a few change their minds and either ring up to say so or just fail to turn up at the nursing home. This would seem to indicate that the majority of women seeking abortion, certainly through Pregnancy Advisory Services, have already made up their minds before seeking help.

It is not difficult to see how crucial the reactions of professional careers are in these circumstances and how much care and kindness the woman needs if her feelings of worthlessness and rejection are not to be intensified.

Case study: a difficult choice about the future

Sarah, an eighteen-year-old single girl, came to a clinic wondering if she was pregnant as she had forgotten some pills and had missed one period. As she was a regular clinic attender with no previous difficulties the doctor asked whether anything was worrying her. She confessed she was confused about her future. She had the offer of a university place and her parents wanted her to go. She was undecided about this — uncertain whether if she did go it would be for herself or her parents, and anyway it meant leaving her boyfriend.

As she had never been away from home before, the doctor wondered whether her anxiety was really about that. She agreed she was worried about this but thought she would be able to cope. She was asked what her boyfriend felt about her going to university. She seemed reluctant at first to talk about this and then said he did not seem to mind though they had not discussed it. Perhaps she was worried about his feelings — the doctor meant whether he really cared for her — but Sarah interpreted this differently. She began to talk about her worries that she would grow (intellectually) beyond him, and felt guilt about this as he was not going to university.

It was suggested that by forgetting her pills even though this was not deliberate and becoming pregnant she was really hoping that her choice would be made for her so that she need not feel guilty about leaving her boyfriend. However, the fact that she had not delayed in coming for advice probably meant that she had mixed feelings about such a solution. (This interpretation proved to be the correct one.)

The pregnancy test was positive. She was visibly shaken and said she did not know what to do. Pregnancy had not offered a solution. She was reluctant to discuss the pregnancy with her parents but would tell her boyfriend and return the following week. When she returned she requested abortion. Her boyfriend was unhappy about the pregnancy but agreed (somewhat reluctantly, she felt) to stand by her. This seemed to free her from her guilty feelings about him, allowing her to think more objectively about going to university. She decided to accept the offer. She had the abortion.

She wrote to the doctor from university saying how she was enjoying university life. She did not regret her decision to have the abortion but blamed herself that it had been necessary.

This case illustrates a number of factors discussed earlier on abortion counselling. Conflict about a decision was demonstrated by erratic use (*not* deliberate) of contraception in someone who had previously taken the pill regularly. Pregnancy was risked in the hope that it would obviate the need to take responsibility for a decision. Added to this was guilt about her success. She thus could not enjoy it and had to rationalise this by saying she was uncertain whether, if she did go, it would be for her own sake or her parents'. Perhaps, if she had discussed this more fully with her boyfriend, she might have discovered that he did not mind her going to university. However, there is the other possibility that she might not have believed him but thought he was putting on a brave face. Pregnancy did not prevent the need for a decision but imposed further painful choices (which is frequently the case). However, it did allow true feelings to be expressed. The clue to Sarah's real feeling about pregnancy was given by her seeking advice early. This was later confirmed by her reaction to the result of the pregnancy test. The self-blame and guilt experienced for allowing a pregnancy to happen and the necessity to have an abortion are often present after a termination.

Not all decisions about a pregnancy are as complex as the above case might suggest. Unwanted pregnancies can occur as a consequence of loneliness and the gullibility and frailty of human beings, as mentioned earlier.

FOLLOW-UP AFTER ABORTION

The community-based or residential social worker is often in a better position to do follow-up than the hospital or clinic worker since women tend to be reluctant to return to the place where they had the abortion. Where the social worker has had a prior relationship with the woman or family, follow-up is easier.

Contraceptive follow-up is also important. There are two schools of thought about when to offer contraceptive advice. Some gynaecologists take the view (understandable since they performed the abortion) that a coil should be fitted either at the time of the abortion or just after or that the pill should be started straight away. The other view is that time should elapse, perhaps weeks or months, before such advice is given.

The professional who already has a relationship with the

woman should advise or help her to obtain advice about contraception. The ideal situation occurs where the family planning clinic doctor or the GP has referred the woman, as they can then do the follow-up as part of supportive after-care rather than as a package deal along with the abortion. If it is offered in a sensitive way, such as by suggesting it might be a suitable time to experiment with methods to see what is best before another relationship is embarked upon, in the case of the single woman, this is usually accepted. Women not unnaturally resent any implication that they are just waiting to hop into bed with the next man.

BENEFITS OF ABORTION

Abortion is so often thought of in terms of failure and disaster that it may seem almost immoral to look at its beneficial aspects. Nevertheless, these may be very real for the woman or her family. Certainly experience from clinic and domiciliary family planning work indicates that the girl or woman who requests an abortion often has a more realistic appreciation of the needs of children. Furthermore, having an abortion can form part of the process of learning to be an effective user of contraception (though obviously it is preferable not to have to learn that way).

Perhaps the main benefit of abortion is that it provides a breathing space or extra time. This may be crucial for the immature girl, or where a future career is in jeopardy or where the relationship is poor. Time may allow the latter to be explored and possibly strengthened without the added stress of taking care of a child. The relationship may, of course, break down altogether. This would hardly have been conducive to the child's welfare. Time may allow health, domestic and financial circumstances to improve.

Abortion may prevent the breakdown of a marriage, which is important where other children are involved. Parents may be better able to cope with and value the children they already have. Abortion in the teenager may enable help to be given to improve the relationship between parent and child. Abortion may be essential for the single girl (Cypriot and Asian) whose chances of marriage would be ruined by a pregnancy. Thus abortion can give people a second chance — an opportunity to review their lives and improve their relationships.

Abortion can prevent the birth of a handicapped child. Ethical considerations obviously surround this issue and only the parents should decide.

Finally, although planned children may become unwanted, and unintended children wanted, nevertheless it would seem preferable to be born without strong doubts about one's birth. It is one thing to express uncertainties about wanting a child during pregnancy, which some women may do, and quite another to actively seek to end the pregnancy by requesting abortion.

PREGNANCY IN THE TEENAGER

The majority of teenage pregnancies occur as a result of a failure to use contraception. As already stated in Part 2, though it is worth reiterating, society does not make it easy for the teenager to seek contraceptive advice. Also, the longer the gap between having intercourse and consciously admitting it, particularly to oneself, the greater the likelihood of pregnancy. A common experience found at Young People's Clinics is that the girl is already pregnant without realising it, when she seeks contraceptive advice. Thus when pregnancy does occur the shame and embarrassment about having sex may lead to statements such as, 'I only had sex once', 'I didn't think it could happen to me' (underlying this, of course, may be anxiety about fertility), 'I got drunk at a party'.

Clinical experience suggests that the teenagers who get pregnant can be divided into three main groups.

Group I: 'Bad luck'

These are the teenagers who become pregnant as a result of ignorance, misinformation and biological bad luck (i.e. some teenagers are more fertile than others and at earlier ages). The girls in this group are not under stress apart from worry about the pregnancy and have good family relationships. They usually request abortion themselves or come alone or with their boyfriend to an agency — the social work agency, young people's clinic — for advice. These girls tend to be more self-aware and with a strong sense of their own identity.

Counselling is usually straightforward with discussion about the circumstances leading to the pregnancy, including the relationship, explanation about the abortion and referral. The girl should be enabled to take responsibility for her sexual behaviour. Contraceptive follow-up is essential. Pregnancy in this group should be seen as one of the mistakes made in the process of growing up, though the pain and guilt involved in having an abortion should not be denied. Also an opportunity for expressing grief and feelings of loss should be provided.

Group II: 'A cry for help'

In this group pregnancy is allowed to happen and is used to draw attention to other problems. These may be within the family, the school, the relationship or the girl herself. The parents' marriage may be going through a difficult patch. They may be so absorbed with this that they fail to notice the distress of their children. There may be conflicts between the parents and the girl about her behaviour, school performance, or boyfriend. Rivalry with siblings may be intensified during the teens. Family relationships that have never been close and affectionate may break down completely at adolescence. There may be stress ignored or unnoticed by parents and teachers. Pregnancy can occur when a relationship is breaking up. Doubts about femininity and fertility can lead to pregnancy though a baby is not wanted.

The majority of the girls request abortion. They allow the pregnancy to be discovered by parents or teachers. They may seek help alone or be brought by parents. Parents are usually angry with the girl and are often only anxious about obtaining an abortion. They may not be concerned about the cause(s) of the pregnancy. The boyfriend, the pill, society, the school or the company the girl keeps may all be blamed by the parents. This reaction may also reflect parental feeling that their little girl is not grown up enough for sex. This in itself may be a contributing factor to the pregnancy. The girl herself is often apathetic and withdrawn.

Great care is needed with these cases since parents, especially where they are responsible in some way for the pregnancy occurring, can easily be antagonised. The opportunity provided by the pregnancy should be used to improve family relationships. When the problem lies within the school the social worker may have to work with the staff, provided the girl agrees. Failure to provide help, which in most cases may be long-term for these other problems, may well lead to severe depression in the girl or another pregnancy.

Group III: 'The need for a baby'

There are many similarities between this group and Group· II except that the girls in this group have decided that a baby is the answer to their problems. Abortion may not be considered. The girl may hide the pregnancy until it is too late for an abortion, or she may present for abortion though in an ambivalent manner, e.g. by presenting late and failing to keep appointments.

The baby is used as a means to an end. As this has already been covered in Part 2, only the main points are reiterated here:

a) to escape from difficult or unhappy home situation;

b) to escape from school;

c) to establish an identity and role;

d) to obtain love and give themselves love and comfort. This occurs particularly in girls from broken homes or who have been in care;

e) to establish independence and right as a separate person;

f) to test the relationship. The decision to have the baby when the partner disowns the pregnancy is often an attempt to retrieve something good from the situation, particularly where the girl has no belief in herself. Where she has a strong sense of self she usually requests abortion when the relationship ends.

The girl needs to be faced with the reality of what having a child, not just a baby (a substitute doll), will mean. This can be extremely difficult since she may only be concerned with her immediate needs and unable to project herself into the future.

Whatever decision the girl makes, whether to have an abortion, keep the baby, give the baby to her parents or have it adopted, she will need considerable long-term support. Giving the baby to mother may seem an acceptable alternative; however, this usually brings problems of sharing and jealousy with the child uncertain as to who is his real mother. If the child is adopted, feelings of loss, envy and unhappiness will have to be coped with. If the girl keeps the child there will be problems with accommodation and finance, particularly if the family refuses to help or there is no family. The boyfriend may abandon her and she will have to cope with that rejection. This may lead her to cling more fiercely and possessively to the child. Later with a new relationship there will be difficulties of sharing both for the child and for the mother. Disciplining by the new father can cause much dissension and a conflict of loyalties within the mother. Sometimes the mother in trying to protect the child does not reveal the true identity of the father. When the child later learns the truth the deception may provoke aggression and desperation to find the real father who may become fantasised into an ideal perfect person. If other children are born to the new relationship, the child may feel isolated and different.

Thus pregnancy in the teenager, particularly those who use a pregnancy as a solution to their difficulties, cannot be regarded with sanguinity.

West Indian teenage girls who become pregnant feature strongly in Groups II and III.

Parental reaction to teenage pregnancy

Mention has already been made of the blame some parents place on the boyfriend etc. Parents are usually angry, hurt and disappointed. The worst that they feared has happened. Some parents pressurise the girl to have an abortion without considering her problems; others, particularly some West Indian parents, may try to insist that the girl goes through with the pregnancy. The parents' refusal to accept the sexuality of their daughter may extend to preventing contraceptive advice being given. Some teenagers may not become involved in a sexual relationship until they are married, but others will. The parents will need help to see that perhaps the wisest policy is to accept their daughter's sexuality and all that that entails rather than risk driving her to deceit, subterfuge and another pregnancy.

Parental consent is needed for an abortion when the girl is under sixteen years. If the parent refuses consent but the girl wants an abortion the gynaecologist usually asks for a psychiatric opinion. Abortion will then be performed if it is considered in the girl's best interest.

Parental consent is needed if the girl is under a Section I Care Order. If refused, the above procedure can be followed. If the girl is under a Section II Care Order the local worker will need to know the local authority's policy in such cases.

The boyfriend's reaction to the pregnancy

Much less is known about this. He may abandon the girl in

panic once pregnancy is confirmed. The girl may fail to tell him. He may accompany the girl to the interview, indicating his full concern and support, or may decide to remain in the waiting room, reluctant to discuss the situation, indicating that he will only help so far.

Illustrative case: Group II — a cry for help

Maureen was fifteen years old. She was the eldest of four children and her mother was pregnant again. She did not know her real father. Her stepfather bullied her, and her mother, to keep the peace, usually took his side. She was doing quite well at school. When she got a boyfriend and started staying out late the conflicts intensified. There were continual rows which occasionally ended with a beating. Her school work began to suffer. She suspected she was pregnant and went to the local social services office. The social worker brought her to the clinic where pregnancy was confirmed. Maureen could not decide what to do. Part of her liked the idea of a baby — something of her own. On the other hand, she had set her heart on being a nurse and realised a baby would interfere with her plans. She was afraid to tell her mother about the pregnancy and accepted the social worker's offer to tell her. During the interview with the mother Maureen said little. The mother, angry and distraught, complained to the social worker about her bad behaviour and how she was always giving trouble. The stepfather joined in and Maureen began to cry. Asked whether Maureen had always been a bad girl the mother hesitated, looking at the stepfather and then replied that Maureen had become naughty after her marriage to the stepfather. Talking to Maureen alone, the social worker learnt of her unhappiness and how the stepfather had always seemed to pick on her and favour his own children. The mother insisted Maureen have an abortion to which Maureen sadly agreed.

The social worker agreed to help but said she felt that as Maureen and the family were having other difficulties it might be helpful for her to come and see them. The mother accepted this, though the stepfather looked displeased. Maureen looked gratefully at the social worker. Maureen had her abortion. She left her boyfriend soon after as he had another girl. The social worker saw the mother and Maureen (the stepfather refused to be involved) over several months. The mother was able to talk about the love she felt for Maureen but how her fear of her husband's violent temper made her take his part. She began to realise how lonely and unhappy this made Maureen. Although the stepfather continued to find fault with Maureen the mother did not join in. Maureen felt she had an ally and did her best not to provoke the stepfather. Her school work improved and eventually she was accepted for nurse training. Four years later the mother and stepfather separated, as a result of his violence.

ABORTION AND MEN

The sexual partners of women seeking abortion are rarely interviewed and much less is known about their attitudes and feelings regarding abortion. Recently an attempt by a husband to stop his wife having an abortion failed when he took the case to court.

Where the relationship is a shallow one or based mainly on sexual attraction, the man is more likely to disown the pregnancy and hold the woman responsible for letting it occur. He may fear that the pregnancy will be used to trap him into marriage and his reaction is likely to be one of panic and anger expressed in the phrase, 'Get rid of it'.

Although there is little documented evidence of the man's feelings, when he does not want the woman to have an abortion and she does, clinical experience shows that it can be equally hurtful for him. He feels rejected along with the pregnancy.

Unlike sterilisation, the man does not have to give his consent for the abortion even if he is the husband. One of the reasons for this is that the paternity may be in doubt. Also proof of paternity requires an elaborate and expensive procedure, which may not be absolutely confirmatory. It is interesting to speculate whether, if the man's signature were required, this would provide a greater understanding of the relationship. However, it is unfortunately more likely that it would lead to delays and exacerbate existing conflicts between the couple. Perhaps if the number of unwanted pregnancies is to be reduced society must hold two people responsible, not just one.

Involvement of the man where possible in abortion counselling both before and after the abortion can be beneficial to the woman and the relationship. Obviously, the man can only be involved where the woman consents.

Case study

A married woman in her early twenties became unintentionally pregnant with the coil. She wanted to have the baby. Her husband did not want the child as he was a student at a crucial stage of his career. They were both from abroad and had no settled home. Reluctantly the wife agreed to have an abortion. The husband appeared greatly relieved. Follow-up was thought essential as it was feared that the wife would become depressed because of her ambivalence.

She returned alone to the clinic after the abortion, complaining of loss of interest in sex and wondered if this was due to the pill she had been given. Her husband was upset by this and they were beginning to quarrel. The doctor wondered whether by withdrawing from her husband sexually she was in fact trying to punish him since he was the one who had really wanted the abortion. At this she began to cry and said that whenever she tried to talk about the abortion he withdrew into his work. It was suggested that perhaps he too felt sad and guilty about the abortion but was unable to talk about it. An offer to see them both was accepted and they both returned the following week. They both looked miserable and this was commented on. The husband then began to talk, saying he did not know what to do. He knew his wife was unhappy and felt it was his fault though they really could not have afforded a child as they did not have a proper home and depended on her earnings. The wife agreed with this. The doctor acknowledged that they both had to make a difficult and painful decision, but thought that instead of denying that the abortion had occurred, as perhaps the husband was trying to do by getting absorbed in his work, they should try to share the grief they both felt. They had lost something — the pregnancy — and they needed to share and mourn that loss. The wife began to cry. The husband took her hand and tried to comfort her. They were seen three more times during which they talked about the abortion and their relationship. Soon afterwards they returned home.

About six months later the doctor received a letter saying that they were much happier and sex was better. The husband had found a job and the wife was returning to college to do a course. They hoped after this to start a family. The wife still got upset when she thought about the abortion, but was now able to share these feelings with her husband.

This case illustrates the importance of follow-up, particularly in those cases where there is ambivalence because of the need to express grief fully. If this couple had not been followed up it is possible that the bitterness and reproach the wife harboured against her husband might have eventually driven them apart. Instead, sharing their grief had brought them closer together and strengthened the marriage. This was achieved by short-term counselling. Had the situation not been dealt with soon after the event, longer-term help would possibly have been necessary.

WOMEN WHO REQUEST REPEAT ABORTIONS

The Lane Committee noted complaints to it from doctors and nurses about such women but commented that these women often have psychological problems with suicide attempts, previous illegitimate children and family breakdown. The numbers are not known for certain. It is possibly 2–6 per cent of all abortions, though the highest number are in the private sector and tend to be among those who are single, in semi-stable relationships, divorced or widowed. There is very little information in the literature about women who have repeat abortions. Brewer (1977(2)) in a study of 50 women having their third or subsequent legal abortion through the British Pregnancy Advisory Service Clinics during 1973–76 found that 23 were pregnant because their method failed, 24 because of erratic use of contraception, and 3 because they changed their mind about the pregnancy. There was a significant relationship between erratic use and a history of medical consultation for psychiatric reasons. There was also a suggestion that unsettled relationships and low educational status were related to erratic use. Of the 190 women having an abortion (82 were West Indian) through the Haringey Domiciliary Family Planning Service during 1968–76, only 20 had two repeat abortions (15 West Indian and 5 English), and only 4 had three repeat abortions (3 West Indian and 1 English) in that time.

RELIGION, CULTURE AND ABORTION

It might be supposed that religion, especially Catholicism, and certain cultural attitudes would be a deterrent to having an abortion. However, this is not borne out by statistics. In hospital regions where there are a large number of Catholics the abortion rates are not lower. 'Catholics are probably not much less likely than other women to opt for an abortion when faced with an unwanted pregnancy' (Lane Report 1974). Cartwright (1970) showed that only about 70 out of 150 — about half the Catholic mothers with Catholic husbands — gave an unqualified negative answer to the question whether a woman with several children should be able to get an abortion, compared with a quarter of non-Catholic mothers.

In the patriarchal cultures where virginity before marriage is emphasised, such as the Greek, Turkish Cypriot and Asian families, if the girl has the misfortune to get pregnant outside marriage the parents will usually insist on abortion if the man refuses to marry her. It has to be done in the utmost secrecy. If it is known that the girl was pregnant she will be unable to get married within her own community. Such a pregnancy is considered a terrible disgrace. Although the religions of these cultural groups are opposed to abortion, nevertheless married women do seek abortions. West Indian women, though individuals may be opposed, also seek abortion when faced with an unwanted pregnancy.

In helping such women their religious views and beliefs must be acknowledged, for while women from all these religious and cultural groups may seek abortion in similar proportion to others, the conflict and guilt experienced may be greater. The ease with which the abortion can be done, paradoxically, may make matters worse and increase the guilt since pain would be a just punishment. If the guilt is too intense the woman may well go and get pregnant soon afterwards to relieve it. This, of course, applies to all women, not just those from a strict religious background.

SUMMARY

Abortion may be an altruistic decision, the result of a confrontation with reality. This refers to those women who have no support, no money, poor housing, enough children or more children than they can cope with already, a relationship that is breaking up or those who do not feel ready for motherhood, or all these things. They have usually thought through the whole situation and while realising that they will feel some guilt and regret about the abortion, see it as the right thing to do in their situation.

An opportunity to talk about their decision, the reasons for it, an explanation of what is to be done and a discussion about contraception may be all that is necessary.

Special care is needed for the young and those who are ambivalent about abortion for whatever reason. Thus counselling is needed for:

a) young teenagers;

b) women with marital/relationship problems;

c) women under pressure from relatives to have an abortion;

d) women who are having an abortion on health grounds or because the child is likely to be deformed, especially where this has been a planned, wanted pregnancy;

e) women who have had a previous abortion;

f) women with a history of psychiatric illness;

g) women who are erratic users of contraception;

h) women who are really asking for help with other problems.

Finally, though abortion is often seen in terms of failure it can be beneficial for the individual woman, the couple and the family.

PART 4
Sexually Transmitted Diseases

16

Sexually Transmitted Diseases

The term sexually transmitted diseases (STD) is now used to refer to all the infections that can be caught through sexual contact or sexual intercourse, including the venereal diseases. Venereal disease is a legal term and includes only three diseases syphilis (the 'pox') gonorrhoea (the 'clap') and chancroid ('soft sore'). Chancroid is very rare and syphilis is becoming less common in Britain. The venereal diseases were defined originally by the Venereal Disease Regulations Act of 1916. This Act led to the establishment of clinics all over Britain where free and confidential investigation, advice and treatment were available to anyone. These clinics (there are over 200) are now part of the National Health Service. Most large hospitals have a clinic situated usually in the outpatients' department. The clinics are usually called 'Special Clinics' though some are given anonymous names such as James Pringle House.

Sexually transmitted infections may be restricted to the lower genito-urinary tract or they may involve other parts of the body, e.g. the eye, by direct contact or indirectly via the blood stream. Babies may be infected during birth in the case of gonorrhoea. Syphilis can be transmitted through the placenta to the foetus. It is extremely rare for these infections to be transmitted by other forms of contact between individuals or indirectly via inanimate infected objects such as lavatory seats.

Syphilis

This is an infectious contagious disease spread by sexual contact. It is caused by an organism called a spirochaete. This can be seen under a microscope but has never been grown outside the body. It can only live in the moist warm atmosphere of the human body and dies within a few hours outside. It thrives in areas like the mouth, the genitalia and the anal region. The disease is divided into three stages:

Primary stage

The incubation period, that is the time between the infection and the presentation of symptoms, is 10 – 90 days. A small painless swelling forms and ulcerates (the chancre) on the site of the original infection. The chancre is full of spirochaetes and is therefore very infectious. It takes about 3–8 weeks to heal. The chancre may form on the genitals, on the anus or rectum (if anal intercourse takes place) or on the lips and tongue (if oral sex occurs). In some cases the ulcer is so small that it passes unnoticed so that the infected person does not seek treatment. In 25 per cent of women the chancre forms on the cervix and hence is unnoticed unless the woman is examined. The diagnosis is made by looking at the fluid expressed from the chancre under the microscope. Blood tests for syphilis become positive after six weeks. Every pregnant woman attending hospital has these tests to ensure she is not carrying syphilis which might affect her unborn child.

Secondary stage

Six to eight weeks after the primary lesions the secondary stage develops. The person feels unwell and may have a sore throat, headaches, fever and swollen glands. These are not helpful for diagnosis. More helpful symptoms for diagnosis are the skin rash consisting of pale pink spots, which cover the chest, back and abdomen, warty growths around the anus (in men) or the vulva (in women) which have flat tops and are reddish or grey in colour, and mouth ulcers, which are small grey raised patches looking rather like snail tracks. The skin rash, the ulcers and warty growths are very infectious. They last for 3–12 months and then disappear. The rash lasts for 6 weeks and affects 30 per cent of cases. It must be emphasised that the first and second stages may be so transient that the person does not realise that he has been infected.

Tertiary stage

This develops from 2 to 20 years after the disappearance of the secondary lesions. Between 30 and 50 per cent of untreated cases go on to the third stage. This is the worst stage with the disease attacking the skin, bones, heart and nervous system. Tumours called 'gummas' appear in the skin. They ulcerate and form large scores, which are slow to heal. Gummas can occur in other parts of the body such as the brain, liver and bones, causing the patient to become very ill. Severe pain occurs if the bones are involved. Syphilis may damage the walls of the great blood vessels, weakening them so that eventually they may burst, causing death. The heart valves may be damaged, resulting in heart failure. The brain cells and the membranes covering the brain can be infected, leading to mental deterioration and eventual madness and paralysis (General Paralysis of the Insane, or GPI).

Congenital syphilis

Syphilis can be transmitted from an infected woman to her unborn baby. This occurs because the organisms multiply in the blood and are able to penetrate the placenta (the after-birth). This takes place from the 20th week of pregnancy onwards, hence the importance of women presenting early for antenatal care so that blood tests can be done and treatment given to prevent the baby being affected. In Britain about 1 in 2,000 pregnant women have a positive blood test for syphilis. About a quarter of the infected babies die in the uterus. Of the 75 per cent born alive, a quarter will die if untreated; of the rest half develop the signs of the third stage of syphilis between the ages of 7 and 15. The progress of the disease in the infant is the same as that in the adult. The primary stage takes place in the womb. The secondary stage is present at birth or within a weeks with skin rashes that are highly infectious. The nose may be affected with mucus patches causing the child to have snuffles. A few develop painful swellings of the bones. In 10 per cent of children infected in the womb the brain is infected leading to convulsions and mental deficiency. If the infant is treated early in life it will be cured, but if it is not, the third stage may develop.

Treatment

Syphilis can be cured if treated in the first or second stages; in the third stage the disease can be arrested. Penicillin is the drug of choice in the treatment of syphilis in all its stages. It is given by daily injection over the course of two weeks for the first two stages, for three weeks for the third stage. Intercourse and alcohol must be avoided. If the person is allergic to penicillin other antibiotics can be used. It is essential that the patient be followed up for at least a year for the primary stage and two years for the secondary stage, in view of the danger of relapse, so that repeated blood tests can be done. Once these are negative, the patient is cured.

Gonorrhoea

This is an acute infection of the genito-urinary tract. It is spread by sexual intercourse. During birth the eyes of the baby can be infected if the mother has gonorrhoea. The germ that causes it is bean-shaped and is called the gonococcus. The incubation period is 2—10 days. Infection passes between the urethra of the man and the urethra or cervix in the woman. If the man is homosexual it can be transferred from the urethra to the rectum of another man and vice versa. As the urethra, cervix and rectum are lined with a single layer of cells the gonococcus penetrates this layer and multiplies. The vagina, being thicker-walled, is not penetrated. The gonococcus is very fragile and dies outside the body; thus it cannot be caught from lavatory seats. Rarely a prepubertal girl may be infected, for example if the girl shares a towel with her parent, and this involves the vagina as it is thin-walled before puberty. Doubt about this manner of infection has been expressed (Burgess *et al.* 1978). Thus sexual assault should always be considered if gonorrhoea is discovered in a child.

Symptoms

Male Usually 3—5 days after intercourse pain is felt on passing urine accompanied by a thick creamy discharge that drips from the penis. If treatment is not sought the infection spreads upwards along the urethra causing increased pain on passing urine. The patient may develop fever and headaches. Without treatment, the prostate gland, the bladder and the testicles may be infected, leading to sterility. Before the days of anti-biotics the urethra during the healing process became narrowed, leading to difficulty in passing urine, and so narrow metal rods (bougies) were passed along the urethra to stretch it. This was very painful.

Female 60 per cent have no symptoms or very mild ones, but they can transmit the disease and act as a silent reservoir of infection. The woman too may have pain on passing urine.

One of the glands near the entrance of the vagina (Bartholin's gland) may become infected. It then becomes swollen, painful and tender. The infection may spread to the fallopian tubes causing salpingitis, resulting in pelvic pain and fever. 10 per cent of women who are infected with gonorrhoea develop salpingitis. The infection may result in sterility. The anus and rectum can be affected when anal intercourse occurs in either sex.

The infection is diagnosed in the male by taking a specimen of discharge from urethra and rectum and looking at it under the microscope after staining. In the woman the diagnosis is more difficult. Specimens are taken from the urethra (by 'milking it' through the vagina) and from the cervix and rectum, then placing these in special dishes with nutrient material. These dishes are then heated for two days. If gonorrhoea is present the gonococci will grow and can be examined under a microscope. Once the diagnosis is made the person must not have intercourse or drink alcohol (since it causes the disease to relapse) and must wash the genitals each day and dry them on a towel only to be used by herself.

Treatment

Penicillin is given as a single injection into a muscle. In most cases this results in a cure, but the patient needs to be followed up after seven days when further smears are taken for examination and culture and the patient passes a specimen of urine for examination. This is repeated three times at weekly intervals. A final check is made after three months. If the patient is allergic to penicillin, other antibiotics are used. This process is repeated for the woman, the tests being done in the first days after her next two periods.

Chancroid

This disease occurs in the tropics and is rare in Britain. Three to seven days after intercourse with an infected partner the man develops one or more small, painful pimples on his penis: the woman develops them on her labia. The pimples grow and then ulcerate. They bleed and are very painful. The glands in the groin become swollen and tender. Treatment is with sulphonamide drugs.

Non-Specific Urethritis (NSU)

Non-specific urethritis has been so called because no specific cause, no organism, can be found. It is a condition affecting men particularly in which the urethra is inflamed (urethritis); the cause, or causes, are not known.

Symptoms

About 10 to 30 days after sexual intercourse the man has a discharge from his urethra which can be clear or purulent. Pain is felt on passing urine. Clinically the disease is identical with gonorrhoea in its early stages, though gonococci cannot be found. The bladder and prostate gland may become infected, causing severe pain. The eyes and large joints can become infected, possibly as a result of an allergic reaction. This is called Reiter's Syndrome; there is no cure. The symptoms usually settle, but there may be further attacks that lead to permanent damage and deformity of the affected joints. About 1 per cent of men with NSU get Reiter's Syndrome. In the woman NSU produces either mild symptoms or none at all.

Treatment

Intercourse must be avoided until all the symptoms have disappeared and for 4—6 weeks after that. Antibiotics such as tetracycline are used. Alcohol must be avoided during treatment and 4 to 6 weeks after as it seems to increase the resistance to cure. NSU is infectious, so partners must be contacted and treated.

Trichomonas

This is an extremely common infection in women affecting the vagina. Perhaps about one million women are infected in Britain (Catterall 1967). It is caused by a tiny parasite, *Trichomonas vaginalis*. It is nearly always transmitted during sexual intercourse. It occasionally enters the urethra and bladder of the female. In the male the urethra is infected but in most cases the man has no symptoms. Infection can result in the woman from splashing in water closets or from a borrowed towel. It can be present without causing symptoms.

Symptoms

Itchy vulva, a discharge and painful intercourse are the complaints of an infected woman. On examination the vagina is tender and a green frothy discharge which is diagnostic is seen. 60 per cent of women with gonorrhoea also have trichomonas. In the man there may be no symptoms, or slight pain on passing urine.

The diagnosis is made by taking a specimen of discharge from the vagina and mixing it with a drop of salt solution on a warmed slide. The parasite can be seen moving under the microscope.

Treatment

Metronidazole (Flagyl) for one week. This should be given to both partners. 90 per cent are cured by one course, the remainder by a second course.

Candidiasis or Thrush

This is an extremely common infection in women of reproductive age, caused by a fungus. It is found in diabetic women, in pregnancy, after a course of antibiotics and in some women taking the oral contraceptive. The latter may be improved by changing the pill. In a few women the problem becomes intractable and they may have to stop the pill. Possibly 1 in 4 women have the fungus present in the vagina, but only 1 in 6 show symptoms. The fungus likes a sugary environment, hence the growth in pregnancy and with the pill (which mimics pregnancy) and diabetes. Its growth is depressed by bacteria, so where these are being treated by an antibiotic the fungus will thrive.

Symptoms

In the woman there is a thick, white cheesy discharge which causes intense irritation. In some women the latter may occur unaccompanied by discharge. The man may develop a sore penis with tiny ulcers that become itchy.

Sometimes the diagnosis is made by demonstrating the fungus on a glass slide. In other cases it has to be grown or cultured.

Treatment

Vaginal pessaries (e.g. nystatin, canestan) 1 to 2 daily for 2 weeks. The man uses nystatin cream.

Genital Warts (other than those caused by syphilis)

These may be single or multiple and are small and rough-surfaced. A number of them may fuse into a cauliflower-like mass ranging from the size of a pea to a cricket ball. They occur, around the vagina, anus and on the penis. The growth of warts in women is facilitated by vaginal discharge due to trichomonas, by sweating and poor personal hygiene. They enlarge during pregnancy.

Treatment

The predisposing cause such as vaginal discharge must be treated. The warts themselves if not too large are burnt with 10–25 per cent podophyllin in alcohol. Several applications may be necessary. If the warts are large they may have to be burnt using electro cautery under a general anaesthetic.

Genital Herpes

This is caused by a virus infection. Small blisters which are intensely itchy and painful are found on the penis and around the vaginal entrance. These blisters break down leaving multiple ulcers which may become infected with bacteria.

Treatment

Washing with soap and water and a weak salt solution will usually help healing in about a week. Alternatively, Idox uridine can be used though the results are not always good. Recurrent infection may occur.

Pubic Lice ('Crabs')

These attach themselves to pubic hairs and eggs are laid (nits). They cause intense itching. Close contact other than sexual contact may result in infection. The lice may spread to other hairy parts of the body excluding the scalp.

Treatment

Gamma benzene hexachloride is applied in the form of an emulsion rubbed into the roots of the hair or as a powder applied by insufflation. One thorough application is usually sufficient. It is not advisable to shave the hair.

INCIDENCE OF SEXUALLY TRANSMITTED DISEASES

The incidence of sexually transmitted disease has been increasing in most countries of the world since the mid to late 1950s. It is difficult to determine the exact number of people affected, as some people may be treated by private doctors who do not report the disease. If these diseases are to be controlled, the names of all infected persons must be notified so that they can be contacted and treated to prevent them infecting others. In Britain approximately a quarter of a million people attend special clinics each year, i.e. 1 in 200 people. Catterall (1967) estimated that of those attending special clinics:

> 22% have gonorrhoea
> 25% have trichomonas
> 25% have non-specific urethitis
> 1–3% have syphilis
> 25% have no infection but attend because they suspect that they have.

It must be noted that repeat infections in the *same* people are reported as *new* infections. Thus perhaps 25 per cent of those presenting at clinics with gonorrhoea are repeat infections in the same people.

Incidence of Syphilis

In England and Wales new cases of syphilis at all stages reported from special clinics fell from 23,878 in 1946 to 3,946 in 1960. The equivalent figures for early infectious syphilis (that is primary and secondary syphilis) were 17,675 and 994 respectively. There has been a slight increase in recent years of primary and secondary syphilis cases, 1743 in 1965 and 1513 in 1973. The latter figure is for England only. (Annual Reports of the Medical Officer, Department of Health [London] [1946–73]

HMSO.) There are conflicting views about the decline in syphilis between 1946 and 1960, whether it was real or due to the gross over-use of penicillin which was used to treat trivial illnesses so that gonorrhoea and syphilis were treated inadvertently. Unfortunately, there is a possibility, due to the dosage used, that penicillin masked the symptoms but did not eliminate the disease.

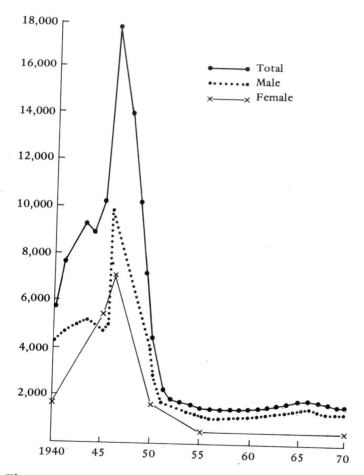

Figure 4: Infectious Syphilis in England & Wales, 1940–70.
Source: R S Morton, *Venereal Diseases*, Penguin, 1966; Reprinted 1972. (Reprinted by permission of Penguin Books Ltd..)

Incidence of Gonorrhoea

Gonorrhoea has now reached epidemic proportions. The World Health Organisation calculates that there are 10 cases of gonorrhoea for every case of syphilis; thus there may be 200 to 300 million cases annually in the world, placing gonorrhoea second to measles. The peak incidence of the war years has now been exceeded in England and Wales. The rise has occurred disproportionately among women under 20. Recent surveys from Western nations show that 55 per cent of all cases occur in people under 25; 3 to 5 more men than women are infected. In the USA there were 270,000 reported cases in 1960; in 1970, 450,000. This is possibly not the true figure as many cases are treated by private doctors and go unreported. This is less likely to happen in Britain.

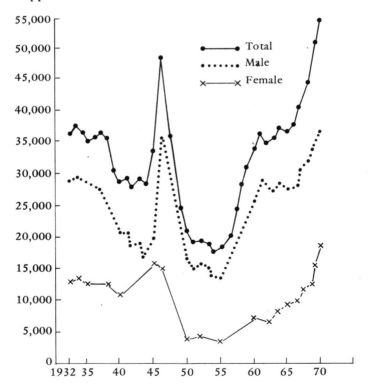

Figure 5: **Cases of Gonorrhoea dealt with for the first time in treatment clinics of England & Wales, 1932–1970.**
Source: R S Morton, *Venereal Diseases*, Penguin, 1972.

Table 8: Number of cases of syphilis and gonorrhoea in various age groups, England & Wales, 1972–75.
Source: Hansard, 27 January 1977, Vol. 924, No. 36, Col. 724.

	Under 16		16 to 19		20 to 24		25 and over		Total	
	Syphilis	Gonorrhoea	Syphilis	Gonorrhoea	Syphilis	Gonorrhoea	Syphilis	Gonorrhoea	Syphilis	Gonorrhoea
1972	8	529	110	9,995	286	18,028	753	24,822	1,157	53,374
1973	8	609	121	11,299	329	19,679	1,055	26,970	1,513	58,557
1974	5	578	143	11,197	378	19,701	1,122	26,545	1,648	58,021
1975	3	552	133	11,755	350	19,732	1,120	26,917	1,606	58,956

Table 9: Incidence of gonorrhoea and syphilis in males and females under 20 years, 1971–74

	Primary and secondary syphilis				Gonorrhoea			
	1971	1972	1973	1974	1971	1972	1973	1974
Males under 20	71	75	86	94	4,522	4,250	4,821	4,772
Females under 20	47	43	43	56	5,998	6,274	7,087	7,003
Total	118	118	129	150	10,520	10,524	11,908	11,775
Males under 16	3	1	4	3	129	109	151	118
Females under 16	4	7	4	2	400	420	458	460
Total	7	8	8	5	529	529	609	578

Interestingly, when the figures are looked at for the 20 to 24-year-olds the ratio is reversed; that is more males than females are affected, possibly because most women are married and involved with child rearing.

Table 10: Incidence of non-specific urethritis

1952	11,552
1958	17,656
1970	47,592
1972	Over 60,000
	(This exceeds the number of gonococcal infections)

Reasons for increased incidence

There are a number of possible factors involved:

1. An increase in population and increased mobility of population including immigration and tourism.

2. Rejection of traditional sexual attitudes and codes of behaviour together with the decline in the double standard of morality. Thus there has been an increase in sexual activity, particularly among young people (though not all the young) which includes girls as well as boys, though perhaps not in equal numbers (Schofield 1965, Farrell 1978).

3. Less use of the mechanical barrier methods of birth control, in particular the sheath, which afforded some measure of protection against sexually transmitted disease. The pill is sometimes blamed directly for the rise in STD. The rise in the incidence of gonorrhoea and non-specific urethritis began in the late 1950s *before* the pill became available. (The pill began to be prescribed in Britain in 1961.) The rise in both gonorrhoea and syphilis is seen in other countries where the pill is not easily available. The increasing sexual activity among teenagers is not accompanied by sustained use of any method of birth control (barrier or pill) (Schofield 1965, Farrell 1978). People under 20 account for 20 per cent of new infections with gonorrhoea (Table 9). One study (Nabarro *et al.* 1978) showed that the incidence of gonorrhoea was very small among single girls attending a clinic for the pill (4 cases out of 1,000 women screened for gonorrhoea). This study seems to confirm clinical impressions and experience that pill users lead stable lives and

have steady relationships, contrary to popular belief.

4. Resistance of some strains of gonorrhoea to antibiotics.

5. Reservoir of gonorrhoea infection in women; 60 per cent of women with gonorrhoea have *no* symptoms.

6. Homosexual men appear to be an increasing source of new cases of syphilis and gonorrhoea. This may only reflect the changed attitudes to homosexuality through the altered law regarding homosexuals, so that they feel free to seek help without fear of prosecution.

KNOWLEDGE ABOUT SEXUALLY TRANSMITTED DISEASES

As venereal diseases were more commonly associated with poor living conditions it used to be hoped that they would disappear, along with other infectious diseases, with the improvement of living standards. However, as mentioned earlier, prosperity brought new situations which aided the spread of venereal diseases. Thus it is now hoped that health education will help to reduce their incidence. Unfortunately, there is still widespread ignorance about sexually transmitted diseases, particularly among young people. Schofield (1965) found that 80 per cent of the girls and 75 per cent of the boys interviewed said they would not have known if they had been infected. Parental contribution to their children's education then was virtually nil. By 1974 the situation had improved somewhat, though less than half the sample of young people interviewed were able to describe the symptoms of gonorrhoea and syphilis (Farrell 1978). What is perhaps more worrying is that nearly half the teenagers interviewed by Farrell who thought they might have had VD at some stage did nothing about it.

Schools are often expected to fill the gaps in information left by the parents. Unfortunately, teachers themselves are often ignorant about sexually transmitted diseases. The Department of Education and Science (DES) has no official policy on sex education. The quality and quantity of sex education is extremely variable. Some schools have proper programmed courses; some just show films without explanation or reinforcement of the information contained in them; others rely on outside speakers. As these diseases are often connected with illicit sex, i.e. pre- and extramarital sex and prostitutes, they are considered 'social and moral diseases'.

They are surrounded by guilt, fear, shame and embarrassment. They are evidence of sexual misdemeanours. They happen to 'other' people (like death and car accidents). Perhaps only cancer is feared as much. Paradoxically, some young males may feel that having a dose of the 'clap' and having survived it is something to feel proud of.

Education about sexually transmitted diseases should not be about horror stories nor used as the stick with which to beat young people. The facts should be presented carefully and unemotionally together with the risks and dangers. The procedure of the clinic should be described together with the importance of contact tracing. One aspect of being sexually responsible is to seek treatment as soon as infection is suspected or risk taken and to encourage one's partner to do the same. Another view of being sexually responsible is not to have pre- or extramarital sex. This is a counsel of perfection which some would find hard to adhere to. While young people have money, access to cars and are unchaperoned, some will have sex before marriage. They should be prepared for the physical and emotional consequences of this. Among the married, couples may be separated for long periods, a marriage may become strained — for example, during the wife's pregnancy — and an extramarital affair may result. The increase in STD is not just among the young and single.

Venerophobia Some patients have venerophobia: they go anxiously from one clinic to another seeking reassurance that they do not have venereal disease. Once reassured they start the process all over again at another clinic. Some of these patients are psychotic and in need of psychiatric treatment. Others are over-anxious as a result of seeing horrific films on venereal disease.

PROCEDURE AT A SPECIAL CLINIC

People may go directly to a special clinic without first seeing their general practitioner, if they wish. At some clinics appointments have to be made. The person is reassured about complete confidentiality. The GP is only informed with the patient's consent. Consultations, investigations and treatment are free. The doctor (a specialist in venereology) interviews the patient in privacy to take a medical history. Then a medical examination is made, together with blood test, urine sample and swabs from the genital organs, rectum anal lesions. Patients should not pass urine for two hours before seeing the doctor, as this makes some tests more reliable. The diagnosis at this stage is presumptive rather than definite. This needs to be stressed to the patient, since occasionally the patient may feel reassured (mistakenly) and hence not attend for further appointments. Follow-up and treatment are discussed. The importance of informing sexual contacts so that they can be investigated and treated is emphasised and contact slips are given to the patient to give to sexual contacts. The sexual contact does not have to be treated at the original clinic where the patient was seen. The clinic where the contact attends usually informs the original clinic of the attendance and diagnosis. There is no moralising or criticism.

The diagnosis of venereal disease may come as a shock to the patient, particularly in a young person or someone involved in an extra-marital relationship. An opportunity is provided to discuss this with the medical social worker (where there is one). Patients who get reinfections often do not believe that they have been adequately treated and so may deny any new contact. It has been estimated that 20 per cent of patients seen in a year will come again within that year.

Some patients default and thus may fail to be adequately treated. There is a higher incidence of defaulting in large cities. People may default because they are careless or over-optimistic, or because they feel guilty about attending a special clinic. The medical social worker has to trace them and persuade them to attend the clinic.

CONTACT TRACING AND THE ROLE OF THE CONTACT TRACER

This is a vital part of the treatment and prevention of sexually transmitted diseases. The special clinics are very careful about contact tracing and are aware of the many pitfalls and frustrations associated with it. This is why it is preferable for the contact to attend a special clinic rather than the GP. Many of the clinics have a medical social worker attached who can offer help both with personal problems and with contact tracing. Medical social workers are selected on the basis of personal qualities as well as qualifications. They have to be tactful, discreet, patient, persuasive and persistent.

The tracing of contacts depends on the voluntary cooperation of the infected patient and this in turn may depend on the skill of the medical social worker.

Contacts are of two kinds — primary and secondary.

Primary contacts

Partners from whom the patient contracts the infection are known as primary contacts. They are often difficult to trace. They may be prostitutes, casual acquaintances and strangers. Alcohol may be a factor in the association so that the patient may not recollect details. Names and addresses may not have been exchanged and so reliance may have to be placed on description. The patient may be reluctant to give details because he may not wish to renew the contact, or he may be ashamed of the episode or fearful of discovery if it is an extramarital affair or the person is a minor. The person may not be able to give all the information about a contact at the initial interview. Several interviews may be needed to build up a picture of the person's life-style and the kind of sexual contacts he makes. All patients must be interviewed carefully because one contact may be known to many people. (A long-distance lorry driver was found to have infected 300 people, and one fourteen-year-old schoolgirl was known to ten young men who attended for treatment at a special clinic.) Where the patient either does not pass on the contact slip or does not wish to do so the contact tracer may have to follow up the contact (with the patient's permission) and explain the problem and try to pursuade the person to seek treatment. An interview may have to be arranged at a local cafe, for example, rather than the contact's home, to ensure confidentiality. The contact may need to be taken to the clinic. Many women contacts are reluctant to believe anything is wrong, especially if they do not have symptoms.

Where the contact lives in another area or has moved, the local medical officer of health is informed so that a health visitor can call. The local special clinic is also notified. In 1969 a society for social workers engaged in contact tracing was formed and a list of clinics where they work was compiled so that they could be contacted directly.

Contact slips have not been found to be so effective with primary contacts.

Secondary contacts

Those to whom the patient transmits infection before diagnosis and treatment are called secondary contacts. These are more likely to be husbands, wives, fiancés and regular partners. Most patients are reliable about these contacts and will give them a contact slip, though this is not without difficulties. The patient may feel ashamed and guilty and fearful about the effect on the relationship. Thus the social worker usually sees all the married individuals who have a sexually transmitted disease in order to discuss with them what to tell their partners. The infected partner is usually advised to tell the spouse that they have an inflammation or infection, *not* venereal disease. Where the secondary contact is the innocent victim it is commonly found at clinics that he/she does not ask straight out whether he/she has venereal disease. It would seem that open acknowledgement that they have contracted venereal disease from their marital partner might necessitate taking action such as divorce which they prefer not to do. Clinic staff in this situation reveal the diagnosis only if directly requested by the patient. Where the marriage is basically sound an extramarital affair can often be weathered. If the marriage is already in difficulty the knowledge of an extramarital affair may force the couple to look at their marriage and try to improve it. The social worker may have an opportunity to help the couple with this either by working directly with them or by referring them to a marriage guidance counsellor. Sometimes the reason for the extramarital affair is the existence of a long-standing sexual problem that has been denied or ignored, and again help may be needed and accepted for this, once everything is out in the open. In other marriages the knowledge of an extramarital affair may lead to divorce. The presence of venereal disease may be used by one partner as evidence of adultery in a divorce petition. The venereologist can be ordered by a judge to reveal the contents of the hospital notes. Fortunately, this rarely happens in practice. Occasionally the occurrence of extramarital affairs by one or both partners forms the accepted life-style of some couples. In these instances they can only be advised to attend for regular check-up.

It is essential with regard to contact tracing that a balance be struck between the control of infection and the freedom of the individual (Catterall 1967).

All clinic staff give particular care to young people attending special clinics, especially the under-sixteens. Confidentiality is respected. Parents and family doctors are *not* informed if the young person requests this, since the staff feel that the young person may not then attend for follow-ups.

HIGH-RISK GROUPS

While sexually transmitted diseases are no respectors of persons and are found among all social classes, nevertheless there are certain individuals who are particularly vulnerable. Some of these will already form part of the social worker's caseload.

The young

While not all young people are at risk since many are not sexually active, there are some who are in especial danger. This may be due to ignorance and/or misinformation, especially among those who leave school early or have been absent from school for long periods through illness or truanting. Sex education, particularly on venereal disease, may not be given until the fifth year, which is too late for some young people. Other young people who are at risk are those who come from unhappy or broken homes or who have been in care for reasons stated earlier — see Chapter 13. Young people who are away from home or who are homeless, particularly girls, may drift into casual sex in order to obtain money for food and lodgings. This may lead to prostitution. Teenagers of West Indian origin are especially vulnerable since they may form a sizeable proportion of those homeless young people in certain city areas. The role of alcohol is particularly relevant to the young, especially young girls. So often they do not intend to have sex but having drunk too much allow themselves to be seduced. (Of course, there are unscrupulous adults who ply young people with alcohol in order to seduce them.) Some young people with low self-esteem lead a self-destructive life-style and take risks with both their health and their lives. In these cases the contraction of venereal disease may be seen as just punishment and may be part of masochistic behaviour. Other young people are bored and have no interests. They may turn to sex for excitement and thrills. By the same token, these young people are most at risk from contracting sexually transmitted diseases and are likely to be irresponsible about using contraception. Thus the girls are at risk from both infection and unwanted pregnancy.

Girls between the ages of 15 and 19 accounted for 12 per cent of all gonorrhoea infections in 1974; a higher proportion than boys of that age. Since more boys than girls are sexually active this would seem to suggest that there is a small pool of highly promiscuous girls.

Subnormal girls

Mildly subnormal girls are at risk because they may be ignorant of the dangers and can be exploited. Some may leave home and become highly promiscuous. They may eventually become prostitutes since they cannot get employment.

The lonely and isolated

People who are lonely, lead erratic lives without regular employment, drift from place to place without close family ties and may be involved with the law are at risk. Men who are away from their families for long periods, e.g. lorry drivers, seamen, are at risk and may pass infection on to their wives or regular partners. Women who live alone with children without a regular partner may be at risk; loneliness may lead the woman into casual relationships with men who only want sex and not the responsibility of a family.

Individuals under stress

Individuals under stress from whatever cause, personal, sexual, marital, family problems or problems with employment, housing, debt, may seek comfort and solace with other partners apart from their regular relationship or spouse and thus put themselves at risk.

Ethnic groups

In the past immigrant men who came alone without their women tended to be lonely and isolated and were strongly at risk of contracting a sexually transmitted disease through casual sex. This is less of a problem nowadays.

Prostitutes

Prostitutes, both male and female, are obviously at risk. The more knowledgeable tend to go to special clinics for regular check-ups.

ROLE OF THE COMMUNITY-BASED SOCIAL WORKER

There is a need for the social worker to:

a) be aware of high risk groups or individuals, particularly the young;

b) be prepared to discuss risks involved, particularly with an erratic life-style, and give information;

c) be prepared to refer and/or take the client to a special clinic;

d) work in conjunction with clinic staff to ensure adequate follow-up to treatment;

e) cope with the consequences — the distress, sense of betrayal — of the discovery of venereal disease, for example by a partner or parents of a teenager;

f) look at and help with the circumstances that lead to the infection, both immediate and past; for example, a sexual or marital difficulty or parental rejection of a teenager.

References

Introduction

Allen, I. *Birth Control in Runcorn and Coalville* F.P.A. Campaign (PEP Broadsheet, Vol. XL 549), 1974

Christopher, E. Should Social Workers be involved in Family Planning? (*Social Work Today*, Vol. 5 No. 20, 9 Jan 1975)

Gochros, H.L. and Schultz, L.G. (Ed.) *Human Sexuality in Social Work* (Association Press, 1972)

Haselkorn, F. (Ed.) Family Planning: The Role of the Social Worker (*Perspectives in Social Work*, Vol. 2 No. 1, Adelphi University School of Social Work Publications 1968)

Kinsey, A.C., Pomeroy, W.B., Martin, C.E. *Sexual Behaviour in the Human Male* (W.B. Saunders, Philadelphia and London, 1948)
, Pomeroy, Martin and Gebhard, P.H. *Sexual Behaviour in the Human Female* (W.B. Saunders, Philadelphia and London, 1953)

Masters, W.H. and Johnson, V.E. *Human Sexual Response* (Little, Brown and Co. 1966)

Chapter 1: Sex and the Normal Sexual Response

Erikson, E. *Childhood and Society* (Penguin, 1965)

Fisher, Seymour *The Female Orgasm* (Basic Books, 1973; pub. in Britain by Pelican)

Freud, Sigmund 'Three Essays on the Theory of Sexuality' (1905) in *Complete Psychological Works*, Standard Edition, Vol. 7, translated and edited by J. Strachey (Hogarth Press, 1955); also in Pelican Freud Library (1975)

Hutt, C. *Males and Females* (Penguin Education, 1971)

Kaplan, H.S. *The New Sex Therapy* (Brunner, Mazel, 1974; pub. in Britain by Baillière Tindall)

Kinsey, A.C., Pomeroy, W.B., Martin, C.E. and Gebhard, P.H. *Sexual Behaviour in the Human Female* (W.B. Saunders, Philadelphia and London, 1953)

Maccoby, E. and Jacklin, C. *The Psychology of Sex Differences* (Stanford University Press, 1974)

Masters, W.H. and Johnson, V.E. *Human Sexual Response* (Little, Brown and Co., 1966)

Money, J., Hampson, J.G. and Hampson, J.L. 'Imprinting and the Establishment of Gender Role', *Arch. of Neurology and Psychiatry*, Vol. 77, pp. 333-6 (1957)

Pincus, L. and Dare, C. *Secrets in the Family* (Faber and Faber, 1978)

Seiden, Anne M. 'Overview: Research on the psychology of Women' I and II, *Am. Jnl. of Psychology*, 133, 9; 133, 10 (1976)

Skynner, R.A.C. *One Flesh, Separate Persons* (Constable, 1976)

Chapter 2: Sexual Difficulties or Dysfunctions

Acton, W. *Functions and Diseases of Reproductive Organs: A Review* (1857)

Bancroft, J.H.J. 'Three Years' Experience in a Sexual Problems Clinic', *Brit. Medical Jnl.* (June 26th, 1976)

Cooper, A.J. 'Treatments of Male Potency Disorders: The Present Status', *Psychosom.*, Vol. 12(4), pp. 235-44 (1971)

Courtenay, M. *Sexual Discord in Marriage* (Tavistock, 1968)

Farrell, C. *My Mother Said* (Routledge and Kegan Paul, 1978)

Friedman, L.J. *Virgin Wives* (Tavistock, 1962)

Gagnon, J.H. and Simon, W. *Sexual Conduct* (Aldine, Chicago, 1973)

Gillan, P. and R. *Sex Therapy Today* (Open Books, 1977)

Hite, S. *Sexual Honesty* (Learner Books, 1974)

Kaplan, H.S. *The New Sex Therapy* (Brunner, Mazel, 1974; pub. in Britain by Baillière Tindall)

Kinsey, A.C., Pomeroy, W.B., Martin, C.E. *Sexual Behaviour in the Human Male* (W.B. Saunders, Philadelphia and London, 1948)
——, Pomeroy, Martin and Gebhard, P.H. *Sexual Behaviour in the Human Female* W.B. Saunders, Philadelphia and London, 1953)

Loudon, N. *et al.* 'Frequency of Self-Reported Problems in a Family Planning Clinic', *Brit. Jnl. Family Planning Doctors*, Vol. 2, No. 3 (1976)

Malinowski, B. *Sex and Repression in Savage Society* (Harcourt, New York, 1927)

Masters, W.H. and Johnson, V.E. *Human Sexual Inadequacy* (Little, Brown and Co. 1970)

Mead, M. *Coming of Age in Samoa* (William Morrow, New York, 1929; available in Britain in Penguin)

Mears, E. 'Sexual Problems Clinics', *Public Health*, London, 92, pp. 218-23 (1978)

Murdoch, G.P. *Social Structure* (Macmillan Co., New York, 1949)

Rainwater, L. *"And the Poor Get Children"* (Quadrangle Books, 1960)
—— 'Marital Sexuality in Four Cultures of Poverty', *Jnl. of Marriage and the Family*, 26, No. 4 (1964)
—— *Family Design* (Aldine, 1965)

Schofield, M. *Sexual Behaviour in Young People* (Longmans, 1965)

Smith, Seymour *Sex and Society* (Hodder and Stoughton, 1975)

Tunnadine, L.P.D. *Contraception and Sexual Life* (Tavistock, 1970)

Warner, M. *Alone of All Her Sex* (Weidenfeld and Nicolson, 1976)

Wright, J., Perrault, R. and Mathieu, M. 'The Treatment of Sexual Dysfunction', *Arch. General Psych.*, Vol. 34 (1977)

Young, Wayland *Eros Denied* (Weidenfeld and Nicolson, 1965)

Chapter 3: Sex and the Handicapped

Craft, M. and A. *Sex and the Mentally Handicapped* (Routledge and Kegan Paul, 1978)

De La Cruz, F. and La Veck, G. *Human Sexuality and the Mentally Retarded* (Brunner, Mazel, 1973; pub. in Britain by Butterworth)

Hamilton, A. 'The Sexual Problems of the Disabled', *Brit. Jnl. of Family Planning Doctors*, Vol. 4, No. 1 (April 1978)

Hilliard, L.T. *Mental Deficiency* (Duckworth, 1968)

Chapter 4: Homosexuality

Altman, D. *Homosexuality: Its Oppression and Liberation* (Allen Lane, 1974)

Babuscio, J. *We Speak for Ourselves* (SPCK, 1977)

Bancroft, J.H.J. *Deviant Sexual Behaviour: Modification and Assessment* (Clarendon Press, Oxford, 1974)

Bell, A. and Weinberg, M. *Homosexualities* (Mitchell Beazley, 1978)

Bieber, I. *Homosexuality: A Psychoanalytic Study of Male Homosexuals* (Basic Books Inc., New York, 1962)

Chang, J. and Bloch, J. 'A Study of Identification in Male Homosexuals', *Jnl. of Consulting Psychology*, 24(4), pp. 307-10 (1960)

Dover, K.J. *Greek Homosexuality* (Duckworth, 1978)

Ford, C.F. and Beach, F.A. *Patterns of Sexual Behaviour* (Harper and Row, 1951)

Gibbons, T.C.N. 'The Sexual Behaviour of Young Criminals', *Jnl. Medical Science*, 103, 527 (1957)

Hertoft, P. in *Psychosexual Problems*, ed. Crown, Sidney, (Grune and Stratton 1976)

Hooker, E. 'The Adjustment of the Male Overt', *Jnl. Projective Techniques*, Vol. 21, p. 157

Kinsey, A.C., Pomeroy, W.B. and Martin, C.E. *Sexual Behaviour in the Human Male* (W.B. Saunders, Philadelphia, 1948)

——, Pomeroy, Martin and Gebhard, P.H. *Sexual Behaviour in the Human Female* (W.B. Saunders, Philadelphia, 1953)

Masters, W.H. and Johnson, V.E. *Homosexuality in Perspective* (Little, Brown and Co., 1979)

Ross, R.T. 'Measures of Sex Behaviour of College Males Compared with Kinsey's Results', *Jnl. of Abnormal Psychology*, 45 (1950)

Saghir, M.T. and Robins, E. *Male and Female Homosexuality: A Comprehensive Investigation* (Williams and Wilkins, Baltimore, 1973)

Socarides, C.W. *The Overt Homosexual* (Grune and Stratton, New York, 1968)

Spencer, S.J.G. 'Homosexuality among Oxford Undergraduates', *Jnl. of Medical Science*, 105 (1959)

Weinberg, M. and Williams, I. *Male Homosexuals: Their Problems and Adaptations* (Oxford University Press, New York and London, 1974)

West, D.J. in *Psychosexual Problems*, ed. Milne, Hugo and Hardy, Shirley J. (Bradford University Press, 1976)

Chapter 5: Sexual Variations

Bancroft, J.H.J. *Deviant Sexual Behaviour: Modification and Assessment* (Oxford, Clarendon Press, 1974)

—— 'The Control of Sexual Behaviour by Drugs: Behavioural Changes Following Oestrogens and Anti-androgens', *Brit. Jnl. of Psychiatry*, 125, pp. 310-15 (1974)

—— 'The Behavioural Approach to Sexual Problems' in *Psychosexual Problems*, ed. Milne, Hugo and Hardy, Shirley J. (Bradford University Press, 1976)

Benjamin, H. 'Transvestism and Transsexualism in the Male and Female', *Jnl. of Sex Research*, 3, pp. 107-27 (1967)

Chesser, E. *The Human Aspects of Sexual Deviation* (Arrow Books, 1971)

Ellis, Havelock *Studies in the Psychology of Sex* (first pub. Random House, New York, 1936; available in Pan Books, 11th edn. 1967)

Freud, S. 'Three Essays on the Theory of Sexuality' (1905) in Standard Edition of *Complete Psychological Works*, Vol. 7, ed. Strachey (Hogarth Press, 1955); also in Pelican Freud Library (1975)

Green, R. 'Change of Sex' in *Medical Aspects of Human Sexuality*, pp. 96-113 (1969)

Hadfield, J.A. *Psychology and Mental Health* (Allen and Unwin, 1950)

Hansard 14 March PQ 0063/1972/73

Lamb, D. 'Follow-up on Ninety-three Patients Undergoing Rehabilitation and Surgery', *Conference Proceedings*, Stanford University (1975)

McGrath, P.G. 'Sexual Offenders' in *Psychosexual Problems*, ed. Milne, Hugo and Hardy, Shirley J. (Bradford University Press, 1976)

Marks, M., Gelder, M.G. and Bancroft, J.H.G. 'Sexual Deviants Two Years After Electric Aversion Therapy', *Brit. Jnl. of Psychiatry*, 117, pp. 173-85 (1970)

Mathis, J.L. 'The Exhibitionist' in *Medical Aspects of Human Sexuality*, pp. 89-101 (1969)

Routh, G. 'Indecent Exposure and the Exhibitionist' *Brit. Jnl. of Hospital Medicine*, April 1971, pp. 531-33

Storr, A. *Sexual Deviation* (Pelican, 1964)

Chapter 6: Rape

Amir, M. *Patterns of Forcible Rape* (University of Chicago Press, 1971)

Burgess, A.W. and Holmstrom, L.L. *Rape: Victims of Crisis* (Robert J. Brady and Co., Bowie, Maryland, 1974)

Gebhard, P.H., Gagnon, J.H., Pomeroy, W.B. and Christiansen, Ov
Sex Offenders (Harper, New York, 1965)

Groth, A.N. and Burgess, A.W. 'Sexual Dysfunction During Rape', *New England Jnl. of Medicine*, 297:14 (1977)

———, Burgess and Holmstrom, L.L. 'Rape: Power, Anger and Sexuality', *Am. Jnl. of Psychiatry*, 134:11 (1977)

Chapter 7: Paedophilia and Incest

Burgess, A.W., Groth, A.N., Holmstrom, L.L. and Sgroi, S. *Sexual Assault of Children and Adolescents* (Lexington Books, 1978)

Cavallin, H. 'Incestuous Fathers: A Clinical Report', *Am. Jnl. of Psychiatry*, 122 (1966), pp. 1132-8

Ingram, M. *Brit. Jnl. of Sexual Medicine*, 44, Vol. 6 (Jan. 1979)

Kinsey, A.C., Pomeroy, W.B., Martin, C.E. and Gebhard, P.H. *Sexual Behaviour in the Human Female* (W.B. Saunders, Philadelphia and London, 1953)

Maisch, H. *Incest* (André Deutsch, 1973)

Pincus, L. and Dare, C. *Secrets in the Family* (Faber and Faber, 1978)

Chapter 8: Family Planning in Contemporary Society

Bone, M. *Family Planning Services in England and Wales* (HMSO 1973)

—— *The Family Planning Services: Changes and Effects* (HMSO 1978)

Butler, N.R. and Bonham, D.G. *Perinatal Problems* (Livingstone, 1963)

Cartwright, A. *Parents and Family Planning Services* (RKP, 1970)

—— *How Many Children* (Routledge and Kegan Paul, 1976)

—— *Recent Trends in Family-Building* (HMSO, 1976)

Clarkson, F.E. *Obstetrics and Gynaecology News* 5.52 (1970)

Freedman R.C., Whelpton, P.K. and Campbell, A.A. *Growth of American Families (Reproduction in the United States in 1955)* (GAF I) (1959)

Heady, J.A. and Morris, J.N. 'Social and Biological Factors in Infant Mortality — Variation of Mortality with Mother's Age and Parity', *Jnl. of Obstetrics and Gynaecology of the Brit. Emp.*, 66, 577 (1959)

Hoffman, L.W. and Wyatt, F. 'Social Change and Motivation for Having Large Families', *Merrill-Palmer Quarterly*, Vol. 6, pp. 235-44 (1960)

Laing, W.A. *Costs and Benefits of Family Planning* (P.E.P. Broadsheet 534, 1972)

Mbiti, J. *African Religions and Philosophy* (Heinemann, 1969)

Peel, J. and Carr, G. *Contraception and Family Design* (Churchill, Livingstone, 1976)

Pohlman, E. *The Psychology of Birth Planning* (Schenkman and Co. Inc., 1969)

Rainwater, L. *And the Poor Get Children* (Quadrangle Books, 1960)

—— *Family Design and Marital Sexuality* (Aldine Press, Chicago, 1965)

Ryder, N.B. and Westoff, C.F. *Growth of American Families (Reproduction in the United States in 1965 (GAF III)* (Princeton University Press, 1971)

Westoff, C.F., Potter, R.G., Sagi, P.C. and Mischler *Family Growth in Metropolitan America* (FGMA Study, 1961)
——, and Potter *The Third Child* (Princeton University Press, 1963)
——, and Bumpass, L. *The Later Years of Childbearing* (Princeton University Press, 1970)
Whelpton, P.K. and Kiser, C.V. *Indianapolis Study: Social and Psychological Factors Affecting Fertility*, 5 vols (Milbank Memorial Fund, New York, 1946, -50, -52, -54, -58)
——, Campbell, A.A. and Patterson, J.E. *Growth of American Families (Reproduction in the United States in 1960)* (GAF II) (1966)
Woolf, M. *Family Intentions* (HMSO, 1967)
—— *Families Five Years On* (HMSO, 1972)

Chapter 9: Fertility and Poverty

Askham, J. *Fertility and Deprivation* (Cambridge University Press, 1975)
Bott, E. *Family and Social Network* (Tavistock Publications, 1957)
Cartwright, A. *How Many Children?* (RKP, 1976)
Cohen, A.K. and Hodges, H.M. 'Characteristics of Lower Blue Collar Class', *Social Problems*, Vol. 10, No. 4 (1963)
Davie, R., Butler, M. and Goldstein, H. *From Birth to Seven* (Longmans, 1972)
Lewis, O. 'The Culture of Poverty', *Scientific American*, Vol. 215, No. 4 (1966)
Miller, S.M. and Riesman, F. 'The Working-Class Sub-culture: A New View', *Social Problems*, Vol. 9, No. 1 (1961)
Rainwater, L. *And the Poor Get Children* (Quadrangle Books, 1960)
—— *Family Design and Marital Sexuality* (Aldine Press, Chicago, 1965)
Rosenthal, G. 'Identifying the Poor: Economic Measures of Poverty' in *On Understanding Poverty*, ed. Moynihan, D.P. (Basic Books, 1968)
Titmuss, R. *Income Distribution and Social Change* (Allen and Unwin, 1962)
Woolf, M. *Family Intentions* (HMSO, 1972)

Chapter 10: Birth Control Services Available on the National Health Service

Adams, T.W. *Am. Jnl. of Obstetrics and Gynaecology*, 89 (1954)
Ambani, L.M. *Fertility and Sterility*, 28, 79 (1977)
Askham, J. *Fertility and Deprivation* (Cambridge University Press, 1975)
Barglow, P. and Eisner, M. *Am. Jnl. of Obstetrics and Gynaecology*, 95 (1966)
Barnes, A.C. and Zuspan, F.P. *Am. Jnl. of Obstetrics and Gynaecology*, 75 (1958)
Bone, M. *Family Planning Services in England and Wales* (HMSO, 1973)
—— *Family Planning Services: Changes and Effects* (HMSO, 1978)
Cartwright, A. *Parents and Family Planning Services* (Routledge and Kegan Paul, 1970)

Chaset, N. *Jnl. of Urology*, 87 (1962)

Deys, C. *Family Planning Association Medical Newsletter*, No. 62 (1976)

Farrell, C. *My Mother Said* (Routledge and Kegan Paul, 1978)

Jensen, F. and Lester, J. *Acta Obst. et Gynae. Scand.*, 36 (1957)

Johnson, M.H. *Am. Jnl. of Psychiatry*, 121 (1964)

Kelsey, M. and Wiggins, P. *Contraception* 9, 11. 15-22 (1974)

Muldoon, M.J. 'Gynaecological Illness After Sterilization', *Brit. Medical Jnl.*, 1, pp. 84-5 (Jan. 8th, 1972)

Oldershaw, K.L. *Contraception, Abortion, Sterilization in General Practice* (Kimpton, 1976)

Peel, J. and Potts, M. *Textbook of Contraceptive Practice* (Cambridge University Press, 1969

———, and Carr, G. *Contraception and Family Design* (Churchill Livingstone, 1972)

RCGP (Royal College of General Practitioners) 'Oral Contraceptives', *Lancet*, 2, 727 (Oct 7th, 1977)

Sim, M. *Brit. Medical Jnl.* (1973)

Thompson, B. and Baird, D. *Lancet*, 1 (1968)

Tietze, C. 'New Estimates of Mortality Associated With Fertility Control', *Family Planning Perspectives*, Vol. 9, No. 2 (1977)

Vessey, M. 'Contraceptive Methods, Risks and Benefits', *Brit. Medical Jnl.* (1978)

——— 'Mortality Among Women Participating in the Oxford Family Planning Association Contraceptive Study', *Lancet*, 29, 77, 2.731 (1977)

Wilson, E. 'Use of Long-Acting Depot Progestogen in Domiciliary Family Planning', *Brit. Medical Jnl.*, 1, pp. 1435-7 (11th December 1976)

———'Domiciliary Family Planning', *Fertility and Contraception*, Vol. 2, No. 4 (1978)

Winston, R.M.L. 'Why 103 Women Asked for Reversal of Sterilization', *Brit. Medical Jnl.*, 2, pp. 305-7 (1977)

Wolfers, H. 'Psychological Aspects of Vasectomy', *Brit. Medical Jnl.*, 4, pp. 297-300 (1970)

Woolf, M. *Family Intentions* (HMSO, 1972)

Ziegler, F.J., Rodgers, D.A. and Kriegsman, S.A. 'Effect of Vasectomy on Psychological Functioning', *Psychosomatic Medicine*, 28, pp. 50-61 (1966)

Chapter 11: Methods of Birth Control

Allen, I. FPA campaign: PEP Broadsheet 549, *Social Science Institute*, Vol. XL (Runcorn and Coalville, 1974)

———*Family Planning Services in the Home (PEP Report, 1976)*

Askham, J. *Fertility and Deprivation* (Cambridge University Press, 1974)

Cartwright, A. *Parents and Family Planning Services* (Routledge and Kegan Paul, 1970)

Christopher, E. 'Should Social Workers be Involved in Family Planning?', *Social Work Today*, Vol. 5, No. 20 (1975)

Mitchell, E. 'Domiciliary Visiting in London', *Family Planning*, 15, p. 107 (1967)

Mortimer, P.J. 'The Probation Officer and Family Planning' (unpublished) (1971)

Oldershaw, K. *Contraception, Abortion, Sterilization in General Practice* (Kimpton, 1976)

Peberdy, M. and Morgans, D. *in Biological Aspects of Social Problems*, ed. Meade and Parkes (1965)

Rainwater, L. *Family Design and Marital Sexuality* (Aldine Press, Chicago, 1965)

Sandberg, E.C. and Jacobs, R.T. *Am. Jnl. of Obstetrics and Gynaecology*, 110(2) 227 (1971)

Smith, S. *The Battered Child* (Butterworth, 1975)

Ward, J. 'Why Do Family Planning Patients Drop Out?', *Jnl. of Biological and Social Sciences*, 3, pp. 301-8 (1971)

Wilson, E. 'Domiciliary Family Planning', *Fertility and Contraception*, Vol. 2, No. 4 (Oct. 1978)

Chapter 12: Contraceptive Counselling

Abortion Statistics England and Wales Series AB No. 2 (OPCS, 1975)

Bone, M. *Family Planning Services: Changes and Effects* (HMSO, 1978)

Brook Advisory Centres *(Characteristics of New Clients at Tottenham Court Road Brook, 1974* (Brook Advisory Centres, 1974)

Brown, G.W. *et al.* 'Life Events and Psychiatric Disorders: Nature of Causal Link', *Psychological Medicine*, 3, pp. 159-76 (1973)

—— *et al.* 'Social Class and Psychological Disturbance among Women in an Urban Population', *Sociology*, 9, pp. 225-34 (1975)

Court Report on Child Health Services: 'Fit for the Future' (HMSO, 1976)

Edmunds, R.H. and Yarrow, A. 'Newer Fashions in Illegitimacy', *Brit. Medical Jnl.*, 1977, 1, pp. 701-3 (1977)

Farrell, C. *My Mother Said* (Routledge and Kegan Paul, 1978)

Finer Report on One-Parent Families, 2 Vols. (HMSO, 1974)

Fromm, E. *The Art of Loving* (Harper, New York, 1955)

Gill, D. *Illegitimacy, Sexuality and the Status of Women* (Blackwell, 1977)

Henriques, F. *Love in Action* (MacGibbon and Kee, 1959)

Hopkinson, A. *Single Mothers* (Scottish Council for Single Parents, 1976)

Hutchinson, F. *Jnl. of Family Planning Doctors*, Vol. 1, No. 4 (1976)

Kinsey, A.C., Pomeroy, W.B., and Martin, C.E. *Sexual Behaviour in the Human Male* (W.B. Saunders, Philadelphia and London, 1948)

Laing, W.A. *Costs and Benefits of Family Planning* (PEP, 1972)

Laslett, P. *The World We Have Lost* (Methuen, 1976)   ·
    and Oostelveen, K. 'Long-term Trends in Bastardy in England: a Study of the Illegitimacy Figures in the Parish Registers and in the Reports of the Registrar-General', *Population Studies, London*,

27, p. 255 (1973)

Malinowski, B. *Parenthood: the Basis of Social Structure in the New Generations* (V.F. Calverton, Samuel D. Schmalhausen Macauley Co., 1930)

Marsden, D. *Mothers Alone* (Allen Lane, 1969)

May, Rollo *Love and Will* (Norton, New York, 1969; available in Fontana, 1974)

Meyerson, S. (ed.) *Adolescence: the Crises of Adjustment* (George Allen and Unwin, 1975)

Pearce, D. and Farid, S. 'Illegitimate Births: Changing Patterns', *Population Trends*, No. 9 (Population Statistics Division, OPCS, Autumn 1977)

Renvoize, J. *Web of Violence* (Routledge and Kegan Paul, 1978)

Richman, N. 'The Effects of Housing on Schoolchildren and Their Mothers', *Developments in Medicine and Child Neurology*, 16, pp.53-8, (1974)
Child Psychology and Psychiatry, Vol. 17, pp. 75-8 (1977)

Ryle, M. 'The Psychological Disturbances Associated with 345 Pregnancies in 137 Women', *Jnl. Mental Science*, 107, pp. 279-86 (1961)

Schofield, M. *The Sexual Behaviour of Young People* (Pelican, 1975)

Shorter, E. *The Making of the Modern Family* (Collins, 1976)

'Social Commentary: 15-25: a Decade of Transition: Building a Family' *Social Trends*, No. 8, 1977; (Central Statistical Office, 1978)

Spicer, F. *Sex and the Love Relationship* (Priory Press, 1975)

Thompson, J. 'Fertility and Abortion Inside and Outside Marriage', *Population Trends*, No. 5 (OPCS, Autumn 1976)

Tredgold, R.F. and Wolff, H.H. (eds) *UCH Notes on Psychiatry* (Duckworth, 1970)

Vincent, C.E. in *The Unwed Mother*, ed. Roberts, R.W. (Harper and Row, New York, 1966)

Violence to Children: Select Committee on Violence in the Family, First Report (HMSO, 1977)

Wimperis, V. *The Unmarried Mother and her Child* (Allen and Unwin, 1960)

Wynn, M. *Fatherless Families* (Michael Joseph, 1964)

Young, L. 'Personality Patterns in Unmarried Mothers', *The Family*, Vol. XXVI, No. 8 (1945)

Chapter 13: Groups that need Special Care with Contraception

Blake, J. *Family Structure in Jamaica* (Free Press of Glencoe, 1961)

Cartwright, A. *How Many Children?* (Routledge and Kegan Paul, 1976)

Cheetham, J. *Social Work and Immigrants* (Routledge and Kegan Paul, 1972)

Clarke, E. *My Mother Who Fathered Me* (Allen and Unwin, 1957)

Henriques, L.F. *Family and Colour in Jamaica* (MacGibbon and Kee, 1968)

Hiro, D. *Black British, White British* (Eyre and Spottiswoode, 1971)
Lannoy, R. *The Speaking Tree* (Oxford University Press, 1971)
Kapadia, K.M. *Marriage and Family in India* (Oxford University Press, Bombay, 1966)

Part 3: Abortion

Birkett Report (of the Interdepartmental Committee on Abortion) (1939)
Breen, D. *The Birth of a First Child* (Social Science Paperback, Tavistock Publications, 1975)
Brewer, C. (1) 'Incidence of Post-Abortion Psychosis: A Prospective Study', *Brit. Medical Jnl.* (1977)
—— (2) 'Third Time Unlucky', *Jnl. of Biology and Social Science*, 9, 99 (1977)
—— Editorial, *General Practitioner* (11th July, 1978)
Cartwright, A. *Parents and Family Planning Services* (Routledge and Kegan Paul, 1970)
Cheetham, J. *Unwanted Pregnancy and Counselling* (Routledge and Kegan Paul, 1977)
Dytrych, Z., Matejček, Z. and Schuller, V. 'Children Born to Women Denied Abortion', *Family Planning Perspectives*, 7, 165 (1975)
Ekblad, M. 'Induced Abortion on Psychiatric Grounds — a Follow-up Study of 479 Women', *Acta Psych. et Neurol. Scand.*, Supplement 99 (1955)
Forssman, M. and Thuwe, I. '120 Children Born After Application for Therapeutic Abortion Refused', *Acta Psych. et Neurol. Scand.*, Vol. 42 (1966)
Goodhart, C.B. *Population Studies, 16* (1972)
Greer, H.S., Lal, S., Lewis, S.C., Belsey, E.M., and Beard, R.W. 'Psychosocial Consequences of Therapeutic Abortion', King's Termination Study III, *Brit. Jnl. Psychiatry*, 128, pp. 74-9 (1976)
Hansard (1) Vol. 950, No. 124, Coll. 711-12, Sir George Sinclair to Roland Moyle (May 20th, 1978)
—— (2) Vol. 953, No. 148, Sir George Sinclair to Roland Moyle (5th July, 1978)
Hook, K. *Acta Psych. et Neurol. Scand.*, 39, Supplement 168 (1963)
Horobin, G.W. (ed.) *Experience with Abortion: A Case Study in NE Scotland* (Cambridge University Press, 1973)
IPP 'Abortion Counselling — an European View', *International Planned Parenthood* (December 1974)
Lambert, J. 'Survey of 3000 Unwanted Pregnancies', *Brit. Medical Jnl.*, 156 (16th October 1971)
Lane Report (of the Committee on the Working of the Abortion Act), 3 vols (HMSO, 1974)
Leiter, N. *New York State Jnl. of Medicine* (December 1st 1972)
Osofsky, Howard J. and Joy D. *The Abortion Experience* (Harper and Row, 1974)

Pare, C.M.B. and Raven, H. 'Follow-up of Patients Referred for
Termination of Pregnancy', *Lancet* 1, 635 (1970)

Peel, J. and Potts, M. *Textbook of Contraceptive Practice* (Cambridge
University Press, 1969)

Simms, Madeleine *Report on Non-medical Abortion Counselling* Birth
Control Trust, 1974)

Simon, N. and Senturia, A. 'Psychiatric Sequelae of Abortion', *Arch.
General Psychology*, Vol. 15, 378 (1966)

Tietze, C. and Lewit, S. 'Joint Program for the Study of Abortion
(JPSA)', *Studies in Family Planning*, 3, 97 (1972)

Part 4: Sexually Transmitted Diseases

Burgess, C.W. *et al. Sexual Assault on Adolescents and Children*
(Lexington, 1978)

Catterall, R.D. *The Venereal Diseases* (Evans, 1967)

Farrell, C. *My Mother Said* (Routledge and Kegan Paul, 1978)

Nabarro, Joan, Grant, A.M., Simon, Rosemary D., Berrall, Valerie and
Catterall, R.D. 'Screening for Gonorrhoea at a Cental London Family
Planning Clinic', *Fertility and Contraception*, Vol. 2, No. 1 (1978)

Schofield, M. *Sexual Behaviour in Young People* (Longmans, 1965)

Further Reading

Titles marked with an asterisk are particularly recommended

For whole of Part I:

Becoming Orgasmic: A Sexual Growth Program for Women Heiman, J.,
    LoPiccolo, J. and LoPiccolo, L. (Prentice-Hall, 1976)
Contraception and Sexual Life Tunnadine, L.P.D. (Tavistock Publications,
    1970)
Entitled to Love Greengross, W. (Melaby Press, 1976)
Homosexuality: Its Oppression and Liberation Altman, Dennis (Allen
    Lane, 1976)
Human Aspects of Sexual Deviation, The Chesser, E. (Arrow Books, 1976)
Human Sexual Inadequacy Masters, W.H. and Johnson, V.E. (Little,
    Brown, Boston, 1970)
Human Sexual Response Masters, W.H. and Johnson, V.E. (Little, Brown,
    Boston, 1966)
Illustrated Manual for Sex Therapy Kaplan, H.S. (Souvenir Press, 1965)
Joy of Sex, The Comfort, A. (Quartet Books, 1974)
Marital Discord Courtenay, Michael (Tavistock Publications, 1962)
My Secret Garden Friday, Nancy (Virago/Quartet, 1965)
New Sex Therapy, The Kaplan, H.S. (Brunner, Baillière, Mazel, 1974;
    Tindall, 1974)
Psychosexual Problems ed. Crown, Sidney (Academic Press, Grune and
    Stratton, 1976)
Secrets in the Family Pincus, L. and Dare, C. (Faber and Faber, 1978)
Sex and Society Smith, M.S. (Hodder and Stoughton, 1975)
Sex and the Elderly Felstein, Ivor (Penguin)
Sex and the Mentally Handicapped Craft, Michael and Ann (Routledge
    and Kegan Paul, 1978)
Sex in Human Loving Berne, Eric (André Deutsch, 1971)
Sexual Behaviour in the Human Female Kinsey, A.C. et al. (W.B. Saunders,
    Philadelphia and London, 1953)
Sexual Behaviour in the Human Male Kinsey, A.C. et al. (W.B. Saunders,
    Philadelphia and London, 1948)
Sexual Deviation Storr, Antony (Penguin, 1964)
Sexual Experience, The ed. Sadock, B.J., Kaplan, H.J. and Freedman, A.M.
    (Williams and Wilkins Co., Baltimore, 1976)
Sexual Options for Paraplegics and Quadriplegics Mooney, T., Chilgren, R.
    and Cole, T. (Little, Brown, 1975)

Understanding Human Sexual Inadequacy Belliveau, F. and Richter, L.N.
(Hodder and Stoughton, 1971)
Virgin Wives Friedman, L.J. (Tavistock Publications 1962)
We Speak for Ourselves Babuscio, Jack (SPCK, 1976)

Chapter 3

Entitled to Love Greengross, W. (National Marriage Guidance Council,
Rugby, 1977)
Human Sexuality and the Mentally Retarded ed. De La Cruz, F. and La
Veck, G. (Brunner, Mazel, New York, 1973; Butterworths)
Not Made of Stone: The Sexual Problems of Handicapped People
Heslinga, K. (Stafleu's Scientific Publishing Co., Leyden, 1974)
Sex and the Mentally Handicapped Craft, M. and A. (Routledge and Kegan
Paul, 1978)
Toward Intimacy and *Within Reach* (on family planning and sexuality con-
cerns of physically disabled women) (Human Sciences Press, 1978)

Chapter 6

Against Our Will — Men, Women and Rape Brownmiller, Susan (Penguin,
1977)
Facts of Rape, The Toner, Barbara (Arrow, 1977)
'How to Help the Raped' Gilley, Judy (*New Society*, 27th June 1977)

Chapter 7

Sexual Assault of Children and Adolescents, Burgess A. W. et al
(Lexington Books, 1978)

For the whole of Part 2:

African Religions and Philosophy Mbiti, J. (Heinemann, 1969)
And the Poor Get Children Rainwater, L. (Quadrangle Books, 1960)
Family Design and Marital Sexuality Rainwater, L. (Aldine Press, Chicaco,
1965)
Fertility and Deprivation Askham, J. (Cambridge University Press, 1975)
Psychology of Birth Planning, The Pohlman, E. (Schenkman and Co. Inc.,
1969)

Chapter 13

Black British, White British Hiro, D. (1971; now available in Penguin)
Capitalism and Slavery Williams, Eric (Andre Deutsch, 1964)
In the Castle of my Skin Lamming, George (Michael Joseph, 1953)
Roll Jordan Roll Genovese, Eugene D. (Andre Deutsch, 1975; mainly
about the American Negro, but also makes reference to the West Indies)
Social Work and Immigrants Cheetham, J. (Routledge and Kegan Paul,
1972)
Family Web Hobson, S. (John Murray 1978; about Indian village life)

Part 4

Sex and VD Llewellyn-Jones, Derek (Faber and Faber, 1974)
VD Explained Statham, Roy (Priory Press 1972)

Useful Addresses

Chapter 3

Blakoe Ltd 229 Putney Bridge Rd London SW15 (for free catalogue of sexual aids)

British Association for Counselling 1A Little Church St Rugby, Warks (for directory of agencies/clinics offering psycho-sexual counselling)

Family Planning Association 27-35 Mortimer St London W1

Family Planning Clinics: addresses available through local Area Health authorities

Marriage Guidance Council (Central Office) Little Church St Rugby Warks

Multiple Sclerosis Society 4 Tachbrook St London SW1V 1SJ Tel. 01 834 8231

Spastics Society Fitzroy Square Centre 16 Fitzroy Sq London W1P 5HQ

SPOD (Committee on Sexual Problems of the Disabled) Brooke House 2—16 Torrington Place London WC1E 7HN (also provide explanatory leaflets)

Chapter 4

Albany Trust 16—18 Strutton Ground London SW1

Campaign for Homosexual Equality (CHE) P.O. Box 427 Manchester M60 2EL

Friend c/o CHE at London office 22 Gt Windmill St London W1; local number published in *Gay News*

Gay Christian Movement c/o 15 Bermuda Rd Cambridge

Gay News mail order 1A Normond Gardens Greyhound Rd London W14 9SB

Gay Switchboards London 01 837 7324; Birmingham, Bristol, Dublin, Glasgow, Oxford, Rochester

Metropolitan Community Church (UK) Flat 3 87 Dunsmore Rd London N16

Parents' Enquiry c/o Rose Robertson, 16 Henley Rd Catford London SE6 2HJ

Quest for Roman Catholic Homosexuals The Secretary 80 South Park Rd London SW19 8ST

Chapter 5

Beamont Society B.M. Box 3084 London WC1V 6XX

Chapter 6

Rape Crisis Centres/Lines (telephone only, except London):
Bristol 22760 Mon. and Wed., 6pm to 7pm
Edinburgh 556 9437 Mon to Fri., 6pm to 10pm; Sat. 2pm to 10pm
Glasgow 331 2811 Mon. to Fri., 6pm to 10pm
London: PO Box 42, London N6 5BU; 01 340 6913 (office);
01 340 6145 (24 hours)
Nottingham 411475 Fridays only, 10pm to 3am

Chapter 8

Area Health Authorities for details of:
local Family Planning Clinics; Psychosexual Clinics; Young People's
Clinics
Brook Advisory Centres 233 Tottenham Court Rd London W1P 9AE;
Tel. 01 323 1522
9 York Rd Birmingham B16 9HX; Tel. 021 455 0491
21 Richmond Hill Clifton Bristol BS8 1BA; Tel. 0272 36657
33 Clarendon St Cambridge; Tel. 0223 55003
Gynaecological Outpatients Coventry and Warwickshire Hospital
Stoney Stanton Rd Coventry; Tel. 0203 412 627
2 Lower Gilmore Place Edinburgh EH3 9NY; Tel. 031 229 5320
Brook Look-in 9 Gambier Terr Liverpool LI 7BG; Tel. 051 709 4558
Family Planning Association, Information Service 27—35 Mortimer St
London W1; Tel. 01 636 7866

Part 3

British Pregnancy Advisory Service (BPAS):
Guildhall Bldgs Navigation St Birmingham B2 BBT; Tel. 021 643 1461;
138 Dyke Rd Brighton Sussex; Tel. 0273 509726;
Coventry Tel. 0203 51663;
Liverpool Tel. 051 227 3721
London Pregnancy Advisory Service 40 Margaret St London W1N 7SB
Tel. 01 409 0281
Marie Stopes Centre 108 Whitfield St London W1 Tel. 01 388 0662

Index

Domiciliary nurses, follow-up visits
179-80
Drugs, psychotherapy uses 53-4,
sexual variations treatment 93
Dysfunctions, sexual 31-69

Edinburgh, unmarried mothers'
characteristics 211
Ejaculation *see* Orgasm, Premature
ejaculation
Ejaculatory incompetence 32,
causes 41, Masters and Johnson
treatment 58
Ellis, Havelock 14
Embarrassment, cause of sex
difficulty 37, of handicapped 72
Emotional benefits of family
planning 127-8
Emotional difficulties, special
contraceptive care 215-9
Environmental approach, social
work 170
Erections 25
Erikson, on psychosexual development 23-4
Ethnic groups, at risk from sexually
transmitted diseases 307
Ethnic origin, and choice of contraceptive method (tables) 243-4
Excitement phase, sexual response
25-6
Exhibitionism 100-1
Expectations, sexual, middle-class
48, unrealised, (case history) 62,
unrealistic 38, young people's
191-2
Experiments, sexual, middle-class
attitude 47, working-class
attitude 49
Exploitation, sexual, mentally
handicapped 76, 223, one-parent
families 204-5

Fallacies, sexual, on intercourse
28-9
Fallopian tubes, portion removed in
sterilisation 158
Families *see* Large families,
Multi-problem families
Families, Cypriot 232-3, West
Indian 233-6
Family, background for paedophilia

victims 113-4, incest treatments
120-1, in Islam 230, sex
behaviour influence 40-1, problems as sexual difficulties 44,
rape problems 106-7
Family dynamics, reasons for
children 132-4
Family planning 124-245
see also Birth control, Contraception benefits 126-9, clinics
for handicapped 74, clinics for
Irish 226-7, personnel shared
care with social worker 177,
religious and cultural influence
225-45, West Indian women's
interest 241-2
Family Planning Association 15,
141, 142, and handicapped 70,
leaflets in Indian languages 230
Family size 126, *see also* Large
families
causal factors 133-4, by ethnic
group and use of contraception
(table) 244, fertility studies on
134-5, immigrants' favoured
225, spacing and limitation 188
Fashion, and fetishism 95
Fear, cause of sex difficulty 37
Femininity, attitude in abortion
counselling 271
Feminist therapy groups 60
Fertility, and abortion counselling
271, control, personal factors
131, and immigrant groups 233,
and poverty, relationship
136-40, studies on family size
134-5, and West Indians 235-6,
240-1
Fertility Guidance Clinic, Dublin
226
Fetishism 95-6, (case histories) 96-8
Fixated paedophile 111-12
Flagyl, treatment for trichomonas
294
Freud, Sigmund 14, on having
children 132, on fetishism 95-6,
on homosexuality 81
Freudian theory 22-3
Friend 86
Frotteurism 102

Gamma benzene hexachloride, for

Injectables, the pill 154
Institute for Sex Research 79
Institute of Psychosexual Medicine
    56, 59
Institute of Sex Education and
    Research 60
Intra-uterine device (IUD, the coil)
    155
    for the blind 222-3, immigrant use
    245, Irish Catholic case history
    227, for mentally handicapped
    223, mythology about 163-4,
    for physically handicapped 221
IQ, sex differences 22
Irish (Catholics), contraceptive
    methods 245, family planning
    226-7, sexual attitudes 51
Islam, family planning 230-1,
    Turkish Cypriots 232-3
IUD *see* Intra-uterine device

Kama Sutra 14
Kinsey Reports 14, on
    homosexuality 78-9, on male
    sexual peak 191

Lack of sexual interest, female 33,
    Masters and Johnson treatment
    58
Lady Chatterley's Lover 14
Lane Committee and Report 248,
    253, 254, on abortion after-
    effects 259-60, on abortion
    counselling 264, on criminal
    abortion 256, on repeat
    abortions 284
Language, barriers for Indians in
    family planning 230, sexual,
    middle-class 46-7, 48
Large families, case history 220,
    contraceptive needs 219-20,
    Roman Catholics 226
    see also Family size
Law, and abortion 249-50, and
    homosexuality 79-80, and
    incest 115, and paedophilia
    112-13, and rape 103-4, and
    transvestism 99
Learning theory, influence on sex
    20-1
Lesbianism 80, 82, 88
Lesions, in syphilis 289

Lice, pubic 295-6
'Like other people' (BBC TV film)
    70
Lippes loop 155
London, Brook Clinic 142
Lonely and isolated, risks from
    sexually transmitted diseases
    307

Macleod, Iain, MP, visits Family
    Planning Association 141
Malleson, Joan 53
Malthus, Rev. Thomas 141
Marie Stopes Centre 142
Marital difficulties, parents'
    contraceptive needs 215-16
Marital Difficulties Clinic 141
Marital therapy 61, for
  ' exhibitionism 101, for homo-
    sexuality 86-7, for transvestism
    99
Marriage, abortion can benefit 276,
    of handicapped 76-7, homo-
    sexuality cure 84, Hindu 228-9,
    Islamic 230-1, in West Indies
    234
Marriage Guidance Council, on
    abortion 259, for handicapped
    74, 76-7, referral to 68-9
Masochism 94-5
Masters and Johnson 14-15, sex
    therapy techniques 52, 56-60,
    (for homosexuality) 85, (and
    the social worker), on sexual
    response 25-30
Masturbation, female 30, in homo-
    sexuality 83, by mentally
    handicapped 75, middle-class
    attitudes 48, for physically
    handicapped 73, 74, working-
    class attitudes 47
Maternal mortality *see* Deaths,
    maternal
Mathematical ability, sex
    differences 21
Medical difficulties 44
Menopause, excuse to stop sex 47
Menstruation, Hindu attitudes 229-
    30, intra-uterine device increases
    156, Islamic attitudes 231, West
    Indian myth 163
Mental difficulties, special contra-

Urine, painful passing, and gonorrhoea 291, tests at clinics 302-3
Uterus damage, after abortion 258-9

Vagina, fallacies removed 28-9
Vaginal examination 55-6, fears of 174, Irish Catholics 227
Vaginal infection, trichomonas, 293-4
Vaginal orgasm, and clitoral orgasm 29-30
Vaginal pessaries, West Indian use of 237
Vaginismus 34
Vasectomy 157-8, immigrant use 245, reversal 158
Venereal disease *see* Sexually transmitted diseases
Venereal Disease Regulations Act 1916 288
Venerophobia 302
Verbal ability, sex differences 21
Vibrators, for handicapped 73
Violence, and incest 118
Virginity, for Asian women 50, for Greek Cypriot brides 232, for Hindu brides 229, for Islamic brides 230
Virility, boys' concern about 198
Visual-spatial ability, sex differences 21
Voyeurism 102

Warts, genital 295, syphilis symptom 289
West Indies, and abortion 285, contraceptive methods 245, families in Britain 236-42, family life in West Indies 233-6, girls at risk from pregnancy 200, illegitimacy rate 206, large families 219, mythology about conception 162-3, sexual attitudes 52, teenagers at risk from sexually transmitted disease 306, unmarried mothers' characteristics 214-15
Withdrawal, contraceptive practice, use by immigrants 245, use by West Indians 237

Wolverhampton, abortion avialability 253
Working-class, family planning service attitudes 144-5, girls and young people's clinics 201-2, poor family planners 136-7, sexual attitudes 46-8
Wright, Helena 53

Young people, abortion rate 195, exploitation of sex in self-assertion 190, contraception special care group 189-204, sexual activity statistics 193-5, sexual behaviour pattern 204, sexual relationships 191-3, sexually transmitted diseases 195, 300, (contacts) 305-6, (high-risk group) 306-7, West Indian girls 237-8
Young People's Clinics 200-2